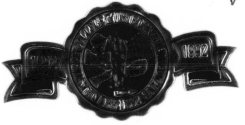

Frontier Doctor – Medical Pioneer

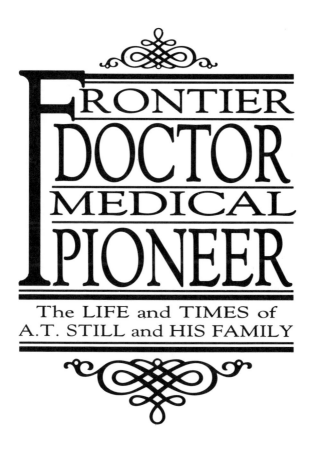

FRONTIER DOCTOR MEDICAL PIONEER

The LIFE and TIMES of A.T. STILL and HIS FAMILY

Charles E. Still, Jr.

The Thomas Jefferson University Press
at Northeast Missouri State University
Kirksville, Missouri
1991

In memory of
Martha Still, Mary Margaret Still, Mary Elvira Still,
Blanche Still Laughlin, and Anna Still

These women faced various hardships with courage and strength, which gave the Still men their courage to pioneer an idea totally new to medicine in the late nineteenth and early twentieth centuries. Without the support and loyalty of these wives and mothers it would have been difficult or impossible for the Osteopathic profession to be conceived, and for a school of medicine established, that is now starting its second century of service.

The Thomas Jefferson University Press
1991
NMSU LB 115   Kirksville, Missouri 63501 USA

Library of Congress Cataloging-in-Publication Data

Still, Charles E., Jr., 1907–
        Frontier Doctor–Medical Pioneer: The Life and Times of A. T.
Still and His Family / by Charles E. Still, Jr.
        p.   cm.
        Includes bibliographical references and index.,
        ISBN 0-943549-13-2 (alk. paper)
        1. Still, A. T. (Andrew Taylor), 1828-1917. 2. Osteopaths–
United States–Biography. I. Title.
        [DNLM: 1. Still, A. T. (Andrew Taylor), 1828-1917. 2. Oste-
opathic Medicine–biography. 3. Physicians–biography. WZ 100
S857S]
RZ332.S85S85 1991
610'.92–dc20
[B]
DNLM/DLC
for Library of Congress   91-797
                                                              CIP

Composed and typeset by The Thomas Jefferson University Press at Northeast Missouri
State University. Text is set in Bembo II 12/15. Printed by Edwards Bros., Inc., Ann Arbor,
Michigan.

The paper used in this publication meets the minimum requirements of the American
National Standard for Permanence of Paper for Printed Library Materials ANSI.Z39.48, 1984.

Contents

Illustrations

Foreword

This is the story of the founding of a profession and of the reform movement in medicine for which it came into being. And yet, it is a family story, charmingly told, in family style. The frontline heroes of the story are men, three in particular: the author's great-grandfather Abraham Still, his grandfather Andrew Taylor Still, the conceiver and founder of Osteopathy, and his father, Charles E. Still. It is so appropriate, however, that the author chose to dedicate the book to five women, mothers and wives who made the heroism and achievements possible. The book is based to a large extent on copious notes, writings, letters, and assorted documents placed in storage more than sixty years ago by the author's father, and on the author's own extensive research and personal observations as a member of the family, as a student in the school founded by his grandfather, and as a veteran practitioner of Osteopathic medicine.

Author Charles E. Still, Jr., asked me to write the foreword to his book because, in his words, of my "judgment and objectivity," supposedly engendered by many years as "close observer" of the profession "from the outside." I find it difficult, however, to be objective about this intimate personal and moving story of tragedy and triumph. Having served the Osteopathic profession and its principles as teacher, researcher, and author for almost half of its entire history, I could not help but find excitement in this saga of the historic and legendary crusade of the Still family for the right to teach and put those principles into practice. Having met the author's father, "Dr. Charley," in the late 1940s, when he was still a member of the Missouri legislature, and having also known the author for many years (on tennis courts and elsewhere), as well as other members of the family, I sometimes feel that I have been caught up in that crusade.

I could not help but feel pride – and a personal stake – in a profession that in such a short time and in the face of enormous obstacles and powerful opposition, progressed from one remarkable man's idea and a one-room school, with twelve students and himself as the faculty, to a profession continually renewed by fifteen first-class medical schools, some university-affiliated and publicly funded, with a collective and superb faculty of hundreds, enrollment in the thousands, and thirty thousand physicians serving millions of patients in all fifty states, as medical officers in the armed forces and the Public Health Service, and as members of numerous governmental agencies, councils, and boards. The Old Doctor is quoted in Chapter 12 as having said in about 1897, when the profession was less than half a decade old, that it was no longer threatened from the *outside*. How much truer that statement is today, when the profession is almost ten decades old!

This is a most timely book as the Osteopathic profession prepares for its second century. Having, in its first century, achieved such enormous success, it would be well for the profession, including its students, to recall its humble and heroic beginnings. It would do well also to remember the noble purpose for which it came into existence, that of basing the practice of medicine on the patient's own inherent healing powers and its support. Having thrived as it has, it would be most appropriate for the profession to determine whether that purpose has also flourished. How well have the health needs that it set out to meet been met? How well are they now being met?

Since the only good reason for the existence of any profession is that it meets societal needs not met by any other, it is timely – even urgent – for the profession to determine whether the need still exists for a health-oriented profession that sees the highest function of the physician to be that of enhancing the competence of the "healthcare system" inherent in every patient and removing the impediments to its function. Given the overwhelming evidence for the increasing need for such a profession, for its preventive as well as its therapeutic value, it remains for the profession to examine itself for what further needs to be done to prepare for this historic role in society.

Were the Osteopathic profession to respond to this book by undertaking this self-scrutiny and rededication to the reformation it began in the nineteenth century, it would have prepared well for the twenty-first century, and the author would have completed his family's "crusade."

Irvin M. Korr, Ph.D.
Emeritus Professor
Kirksville College of Osteopathic Medicine, 1975
Texas College of Osteopathic Medicine, 1990

Fort Worth, Texas
April 1991

Acknowledgments

I congratulate my father, **Dr. Charley Still**, for providing so much material in his notes on the life of his father, Andrew Taylor Still, and on the early history of the school and the Osteopathic profession. No other person was in a better position to chronicle the events so well. I hope that I have used his unedited notes, his collection of letters, and my recollection of our conversations to paint an accurate picture of the life and times of Andrew Taylor Still and his family.

I am especially grateful to **Eleanor Ninmam-Schultz** whose astute editorial work – and editor's red pencil – helped eliminate meanderings, repetition, and caught some factual inaccuracies. Her editorial work and long hours resulted in the final manuscript.

My thanks extends to others who have assisted me in this project. Elizabeth Laughlin was the motivator, ever ready to provide pictures, genealogical material, and additional information. She also encouraged me when I needed it most. Nadine Smith, my writing instructor at Scottsdale (Arizona) Community College, helped me learn the basics of writing. She also read the unfinished manuscript and gave suggestions and encouragement. Ken Bacher, my manuscript consultant, guided me through the eighteen chapters, advising me and correcting a variety of mixed-up sentences. I thank him for his sincere interest in the project. Mark Laughlin carefully read every page when it was in the roughest condition, making constructive suggestions and offering words of encouragement.

Inspiration was gained from the following published sources: and my grandfather's *Autobiography* (1897); E. R. Booth's *History of Osteopathy and Twentieth-Century Medicine* (1905); Arthur G. Hildreth's *The Lengthening Shadow of Dr. Andrew Taylor Still* (1938); and Georgia Walter's "The First School of Osteopathy," in The Kirksville Magazine. By way of honoring my father, I have appended to chapter eighteen a tribute to "Dr. Charley" written by Dr. William Englehard in 1936 for *The Journal of Osteopathy*.

Finally, this project would not have been complete without the cooperation of Kirksville College of Osteopathic Medicine, the A. T. Still National Osteopathic Museum, and Northeast Missouri State University.

Preface

During the years I have been returning to Kirksville to attend post-graduate classes and Founder's Day celebrations, I have talked to many former students of the college. Among them were a few who knew something about the history of their profession and the life of its founder; however, they were definitely in the minority. Most of them knew little of the life of Andrew T. Still, of his parents, or of other family members who had done so much to help the Osteopathic profession during its early period of growth and the many rough times it experienced as it matured. Hardly any of the graduates knew about the contributions of friends of the profession in its early days or how the zeal and enthusiasm of the first graduates insured both the growth and prestige of their profession.

My father, Dr. Charley, at one point planned to write a book about his father's life and the early history of the college, and in 1924 and 1925, he gathered material for the manuscript. He had written to a large number of the college's graduates asking them to relate their experiences at the school and their thoughts and feelings about the Old Doctor. In all, he received more than forty letters in response.

During that same time period, about once a week he would dictate a page or two of remembrances of his father, the beginning of the school, and his own experiences as the first person – other than his father – to go into the world and practice Osteopathy. However, he soon became involved in so many other activities that he never got around to writing his book. As a result, some twenty years later he presented all of his material to me and my sister, Elizabeth. He asked us if, sometime in the future, we could see that this material would be used in preparation of a book.

A little more than five years ago, after having practiced Osteopathy for fifty years, I dug out the metal box in which Dad had placed the letters and his own writings. They had been stored away for more than sixty years. Unfortunately, he had taken all of his letters out of their envelopes. As a result, in many cases quite a few pages have been lost or torn, including the last pages with the signatures. Unless letters had been written on pages with letterheads, it was impossible to be sure of the names of the writers.

Since I had retired and had some time, one of my first cousins by marriage, Elizabeth Laughlin, insisted that I try to do something with this material so my father's efforts would not be lost. After looking over the contents of the box, I would have been more than happy to forget about this project. It was truly a mess. My cousin was persistent, however, noting that I had spent the first ten and one-half years of my life living next door to my grandfather and I was therefore the logical one to write a book about his life and about the life of his family, as well. Elizabeth also pointed out that I was raised next door to the hospital and less than a block from the infirmary, and that I had seen quite a bit of the growth of the school and the profession firsthand.

I had been exposed to my father's experiences and also had heard Uncle Harry Still, Aunt Blanche Laughlin, and Uncle Herman Still (who lived with us the last fifteen years of his life), discuss their early lives and the profound impact that all of the difficult years at the start of the Osteopathic profession had made on all the family. I had been truly fortunate to know all the members of Andrew Still's immediate family and to hear them give so much credit to their mother for her part in launching this new profession. I had also had the opportunity to know my Uncle George Laughlin well. He later headed the college in Kirksville. In addition, on several occasions I had the chance to spend some time with my mother's brother, Uncle Bob Rider.

In the end, cousin Elizabeth was so persuasive that I decided to write this book on the family history, using my father's notes. Once I had reached a firm decision to write the book about my family in general and my grandfather in particular, I felt that I needed as much information as possible in addition to family members' discussions and writings. Although there were already several books on Andrew Still's life, I felt that I had better do a little digging of my own.

First I went to Jonesville, Virginia, where Andrew Still was born; then on to New Market, Tennessee, where the family lived for a while. As I followed the family's trail through Missouri, on to Kansas, and then back to Missouri, it was necessary to dig through the archives and historical collections of the libraries at the University of Kansas in Lawrence, the University of Missouri in Columbia, and Baker University in Baldwin City, Kansas. I found additional material about Andrew's life and times in reports from county historical societies and in the archives of the states of Kansas and Missouri. From a historical standpoint, the pre-Civil War period was one of the most exciting times in the growth of our nation, and the Still family was deeply involved in the action.

As far as the development of the profession was concerned, it was necessary to use much of my own information from discussions with my father and from his writings. I am sorry I was not able to give more space, which was so richly deserved, to the accomplishments of other family members and many pioneers of the profession.

I was very fortunate to have the opportunity to spend some time with Dr. Carl McConnell, an Osteopathic writer and researcher, during the last months of his life. Although he was dying, we had several long and thought-provoking discussions.

Dr. McConnell pointed out that he was more convinced than ever that the mechanical factor, as a major causative factor in the development of disease, had been only partly explored. He felt it necessary to evaluate all factors to really understand the underlying cause of heart attacks. He said he felt there were several mechanical components that affected the arterial circulation of the blood vessels of the heart and that when they were found and evaluated we would have a better understanding of the causes of heart malfunction. He was still working on this concept at the time of his death.

Dr. McConnell was only one of many whom I have been privileged to know who still had enthusiasm and dedication to the profession and its concepts after practicing Osteopathy exclusively for forty years or more. Many felt that this dedication to the principles of their profession was the major reason for the continued growth of Osteopathy as an independent school of medicine.

I hope that I have been able to present Andrew Still, his family, and the profession in an interesting and readable fashion. Andrew Still had a full, useful, and exciting life. There was considerable conflicting source material, and often there were various dates for specific events in his life. The chronology was often confusing and there are still some controversies that are unresolved. Nevertheless, I have tried to be as accurate as possible and have strived to be as objective as possible.

Having again savored the enthusiasm of Osteopathy's early years, I still feel that our potential for both service and growth lies ahead. Maybe we should take the Old Doctor's advice: "Strap on some enthusiasm, and dig on!"

Charles E. Still, Jr.

Scottsdale, Arizona
March 1991

Chapter One

MARTHA STILL WAS FURIOUS. It was the second day in a row that young Andrew had come home with raw areas and bruises on his legs from a thrashing he had gotten from his teacher at the log cabin schoolhouse. What made Martha even angrier was that not only were her children being punished regularly and rather brutally but they were learning so little.

Ed and Jim, her two older sons, had also complained about the harsh treatment at school. Recently the teacher seemed to have lost control of his temper completely and the beatings were becoming even more severe.

Martha was a frontier woman, and she used a switch on her children when they needed it. But senseless whipping could not be tolerated. She had often discussed the school situation with her husband whenever he was home. She urged him to think about moving someplace where she might get her children a better education and where they might also be away from this teacher with the uncontrollable temper.

It wasn't that she didn't like their home. She loved the small farm that was just a few miles from the little town of Jonesville in Lee County in southwestern Virginia. Furthermore, the Blue Ridge Mountains to the south of their log cabin were always an inspiration to her. The twisted trail that led through the mountains was impassable by wagons and later earned the name "trail of the lonesome pine," because it could be crossed only by foot or by an expert horseman.

1

Martha had married Abram Still in 1822, two years before he became a circuit riding preacher for the new and expanding Methodist Church. These new preachers on horseback, with only their Bibles in hand, were the unique development of the church in 1783. Shortly thereafter, Methodist Camp Meetings developed where hundreds of worshipers would gather for several days at a time to hear preaching and sing hymns.

Martha remembered vividly how she met Abram. It was at one of those Camp Meetings when many young men were inspired with such religious fervor and zeal that they all wanted to become circuit riding preachers.

At first, only unmarried men were accepted for this lonely and demanding assignment, but this soon changed. Because of the rigorous work, the wearying weeks of riding horseback, no assurance of a place to sleep, and no protection from the weather, many of the men became discouraged and dropped out after a few months.

But circuit riding was truly Abram's life. With no church buildings in which to preach, each mountain cabin was a place to deliver his spontaneous sermons. As lonely, as physically and mentally draining as his work was, Abram faced each day with a feeling of joy. He exulted in the fact that he could bring the word of God to so many isolated families.

Nonetheless, after six weeks on horseback and traveling from cabin to cabin, family to family, it was always a relief to have a wife and home to return to for some much needed rest. But even as he relaxed and restored his strength, he knew that soon he would be anxious to get back to his assignment again.

The Holston Conference of the Methodist Church operated in an area characterized by small farms and isolated families, often far from civilization, and deep in the mountains. Before long, circuit riding preachers brought back word that many families they visited had serious physical problems and often needed medical attention.

Quite a few of the preachers took it upon themselves to study and learn as much as they could about how to minister to the sick. Abraham was one of them. He soon developed the knowledge and skill to take care of many of the physical problems and ills even as he tended to the spiritual health of the isolated families. As he continued his ministrations, he felt he was now even more useful to the church and to the people because he was serving both the body and the spirit.

He realized for some time that Martha was not happy with the school situation in Jonesville. In addition, he knew their small log cabin was hardly large enough for their growing family that now included five children. When Martha asked him seriously to see if they might move someplace where the children could get a better education – one of her primary interests for their children – he contacted the Methodist Church Conference headquarters.

He was told the church was planning to build a school at New Market, Tennessee and he could be assigned to that project if he wished. At first he was a bit reluctant. Though he wanted to grant Martha's wish, he didn't really want to move away from families he had served, and he didn't want to leave the lovely Blue Ridge Mountains. Yet, Abraham was a man who liked a challenge, and this would give him a chance to add new direction to his life. It would also give his children the opportunity to gain the education Martha wanted for them. So Abraham accepted this new position, knowing his family would be a lot happier.

That summer, after the children had helped in the house and all the farm chores were done, Martha loaded the family into the largest wagon the family owned. They rode to nearby Jonesville where Martha spent several hours picking up supplies for the family's move to Tennessee.

It was usually during the summer that wagons and carts, drawn by horses and oxen, stopped in Jonesville for supplies as families traveled through the Cumberland Gap and on to the West. The youngsters – Ed, Jim, and "Drew" (Andrew's nickname) – watched with excitement and a degree of envy as those families loaded their wagons with fresh supplies and headed on to the West. Even Barbara Jane, who was only four years old, was excited by this activity, understanding that soon they, too, would head West to find a new home.

Abraham and Martha, with the five children and all their possessions loaded into two ox-drawn wagons, finally began the trip to New Market, a journey that would take nearly a month. The youngest child, Thomas, was only a year old at the time.

Along the way, Martha had plenty of time to think about her life – its past, and what she expected of the future. She remembered stories her father told of his family's adventures. How his father, James Moore III, and his aunt had been captured by Shawnee Indians and were later sold in Canada as slaves; how the rest of his family had been killed by the same tribe near the small Virginia community of Abb's Valley; and how it took her grandfather, with his sister, several years to escape from their captors. (These relatives were Martha's grandfather and great-aunt.) After her grandfather's return to Virginia, he started a family on a small farm in Tazewell County, Virginia. Her father followed in the family tradition and also became a farmer.

Undoubtedly, Martha's great concern for her children to get an education was inspired by the fact that she had been unable to get a formal education herself since the only available school at that time was for men only. She learned to read, however, and spent much of her time reading when not helping with family chores. This prompted her to resolve that, whatever else happened, she would see that her children had every opportunity to attend a school.

EVEN WITH THE SLOWNESS of the trip in the wagons behind the plodding oxen, Martha's spirits soared. Her dream of a good education for her children, she believed, would now be fulfilled. When they arrived at their destination and she saw the family's new home in New Market, Martha was truly happy. There was a well-kept front yard and a small vegetable garden. Best of all, it was a frame house with several rooms. As she helped unload the wagons, she felt that at last her family would have the opportunities that she had so wished for it: a nice home with a good school nearby.

Abraham had also done a lot of thinking during this trip to his new assignment. The Conference leaders had told him he was to help build and develop the new school and he would also be allowed to preach. He could not help but assume that preaching down in the lowlands might be a bit different from his work with the mountain families in their lonely cabins.

Although he had some doubts about this assignment, he was glad that he would be near Knoxville where, he had heard, there were really fine doctors. He decided that if the opportunity came he would gain additional medical knowledge. One thing he hadn't thought much about was that many of these farms had slaves. He knew his father, Boaz, owned a large farm near Asheville in Buncombe County, North Carolina, and had blacks help on the farm; but at his young age, he hadn't thought of them as slaves.

Most of the farms in the mountain area where Abraham had first been stationed were too small to use more help, and at no time had the slavery issue been a problem for him or for many other circuit riding preachers serving that area. He knew that none of his friends or associates owned slaves, and most of them were opposed to the idea, but here on the flatland nearly all the farmers with considerable property owned slaves and many treated them with little or no consideration – some in a very inhumane, even cruel, manner.

So Abraham had much to ponder as he began his new position. Would he be able to accept the different treatment of human beings simply because of the color of their skin? Other preachers seemed to be comfortable with such a situation, but not Abraham. He began to doubt whether he could live with himself if he didn't speak up against slavery.

During the ten years he had served as a circuit rider in the mountains of southwestern Virginia he had established such a fixed life-style that he found it quite difficult to make what was a dramatic and radical change in his work and daily routine. When he heard that one of his younger brothers, Elijah, was now serving as a circuit riding preacher to the mountain families in Tazewell County, one of the most mountainous regions in the whole state of Virginia, Abraham felt a twinge of envy. He missed all those lovely mornings when he watched the sun burn the mist off of his beautiful Blue Ridge Mountains. Now they seemed so far away.

There were other changes in Abraham's work that he had not anticipated. He wasn't preaching as often as he had in the past, nor was it to isolated families. He found that the small churches and their congregations expected a much different type of presentation. They wanted a properly prepared sermon, but Abraham was used to speaking extemporaneously.

With his zeal for his church and its growth, he felt he must spend more of his time becoming forceful and eloquent. Other preachers shared some of his feelings about the evils of slavery, but they were careful to keep their opinions on the subject to themselves.

The fine brick school, sitting on a hill overlooking the small town of New Market, was finished shortly before the

Still family moved into their new home. (Later, during the War Between the States, the school would be badly damaged.)

THE SCHOOL SERVED the Methodist farm families in the surrounding area. Operated by the Holston Conference, it was called Holston College or Academy, but it served only as an elementary and secondary school. The Conference was fortunate to have selected Henry Saffel, a dedicated educator, to head the school because he emphasized sound basic courses and he carefully supervised the quality of the teaching offered in the classes. The Still boys – Ed, Jim, and Andrew – were exposed for the first time to a real opportunity to learn.

Martha felt a true sense of security when the Conference appointed her husband to serve, along with his other assignments, as the agent for Holston College. His new job would require contacting potential students as well as raising funds so the school could grow. With a nice home near a good school, Martha felt she now had the ideal situation in which to raise her ever-expanding family. Finally, there would be stability in her life.

During February of 1836, John Wesley Still was born. Martha and Abraham now had five boys and one girl. Martha's only unsolved problem was that, thus far, the school had made no provision for female students. However, there were several good teachers available who would teach her daughter, Barbara Jane.

Martha had been so absorbed in her own interests that she failed to notice how restless Abraham had become. She knew that he was busy most of the time and, usually, if he were active enough, he was happy.

For some time Abraham had felt less enthused about his work and his life in general. He was now so taken up with contacting prospective students and raising money for the school, not only from the farm families but from the administrative leaders of the Holston Conference, that he had less and less time to preach. Maybe some of his sermons had had too strong an antislavery tone because his preaching assignments had been greatly reduced.

Most of all, Abraham missed being on horseback, riding through the land visiting the widely scattered families and bringing them the word of God. He knew that these people would otherwise have been deprived of hearing a sermon given in their homes. He considered his main mission in life was to preach on a one-to-one basis and to pray with these families.

With dedication and eagerness to expand the growth of the Methodist Church and to be true to what he could do best, he conferred with the leaders of the church. When they said they wanted him to spread Methodism to the sparsely populated areas of northern Missouri and that he would be opening up a brand new territory, he readily accepted their proposal.

Actually, the Methodist Church had expanded into the southern part of Missouri nearly twenty years earlier when its first church was established in Cape Girardeau. A year or two later, several more churches had been located in the southeastern part of the state, as well as one in the growing city of Saint Louis. At this time, however, the northern area was still virgin territory for the expansion of Methodism.

Once again Abraham would be doing what he loved best: being a circuit rider. He felt this was a great challenge, one that his wife and children would be happy to help him meet.

Martha was the loyal wife of a circuit rider. She knew that although she might hope for stability, there was always the good possibility of a sudden move – such as the one facing her now. She certainly would not have chosen to go to such a sparsely populated area where there were no schools, churches, or stores. As she planned for the long trip, she tried to prepare herself mentally and emotionally to join in the enthusiasm of her children and husband in what they anticipated as an exciting new experience.

The boys had heard about all of the wild game to hunt and Ed, now age thirteen, had heard about all the good farmland that would be available when he was able to strike out for himself.

The Conference had given Abraham seven hundred dollars for his first year in the new territory and seven horses to pull his two wagons. The trip across Tennessee during the early summer was quite pleasant; neither too hot nor too cold. There was very little rain and they crossed the rivers of Tennessee with little or no problem.

The family had heard about the steamboats on the mighty Mississippi, so when the wagons neared the river everyone's excitement reached a fever pitch. As they came to a point about two miles from the river, a short distance from Cairo, Illinois, they heard a deep-throated blast. Abraham had a hard time controlling the boys as well as the horses. The boys wanted to whip the horses so they could get an even quicker view of a steamboat. Standing on the riverbank, they marveled as the largest moving object they had ever seen went steaming by. It was going upstream, its smokestack belching black columns into the cloudless sky. The boat was close enough for the boys to see the passengers, as well as the horses, cattle, and bales of cotton. They stood in awe until the boat disappeared upriver.

The Ohio River's confluence with the Mississippi is near Cairo, so the family doubled back to the ferry crossing after their exciting first view of a steamboat. When they boarded the horse-drawn ferryboat, the Ohio looked almost as wide to them as the Mississippi. That night, they set up camp on the Illinois side. The next morning, as they started north along the east bank of the Mississippi River, the weather – which had been so nice – turned into heavy summer rains, transforming the road into a quagmire.

For the next twelve days, their two wagons wallowed through one mud hole after another. The black Illinois mud was deeper and stickier than anything they had ever encountered and they often had to hire a pilot to help them avoid the deeper holes.

There were times, even when the rains weren't quite so heavy, that the mud holes seemed to have an excess of water. Abraham began to believe that some of the farmers were adding extra water to the holes so they could make money by hitching up their mules and pulling unfortunate travelers out of the apparently well-cultivated mud holes. He may have been right, for tradition has it that this became a standard method of earning extra income, continuing until the last of those roads was paved in the twentieth century.

The boys spent most of their time standing knee-deep in mud, pushing the wagons toward the Mississippi River crossing. By the time the Still wagons had reached a place on the river opposite Saint Louis, the wagons, horses, and most of the family were caked with black Illinois soil. The trip across the river on a steam-driven ferry gave the boys another new experience, their first opportunity to see a steam engine in operation at close range.

Upon their arrival in Saint Louis, Abraham looked up the resident Methodist minister and the family was invited to attend his services on the following Sunday. It took nearly two days to get the caked mud off the horses and wagons, and the children needed several scrubbings before they were allowed to put on their Sunday clothes.

By the time Sunday arrived, Martha had spent three days washing and rewashing the clothes the family had worn during the trip. By the time church started on Sunday, all the scrubbing and soap and water had produced six clean children who, along with their parents, were seated in the front row of the Saint

Louis Methodist Church and raptly listening to an inspiring sermon by Rev. Harmon.

Rev. Harmon so impressed Abraham that when the preacher asked to borrow some money for a couple of months, Abraham loaned him the entire seven hundred dollars that the Conference had given him for his first year's existence in northern Missouri!

When the Stills left Saint Louis, the weather was again nearly perfect for the trip north to Macon County. They saw very few people, and the scenery was mostly empty grassland. The roads were narrow and poorly marked and a few times they discovered themselves lost, with no one around to give them directions.

By the time they reached Macon County, they had experienced some cool nights that indicated the arrival of an early autumn. It was only after they started looking for a place to spend their first year in Missouri that Martha learned Abraham had loaned all of his seven hundred dollars to the preacher in Saint Louis. She had saved a little more than three hundred dollars over the years, and it took nearly all of her savings just to pay for their housing needs.

Even before they moved into their new home and before the wagons were completely unloaded, Abraham was on horseback, off doing what he loved so much: riding to isolated farm families, bringing the word of God to northern Missouri.

Being the first Methodist preacher in this area brought a real sense of pride to Abraham. He was now serving under the jurisdiction of the Missouri Conference. Over the next six years he was assigned to five different circuits: Macon, Goshen, Waterloo, Edina, and Spring Creek. As a dedicated circuit rider, he followed the same pattern he had established many years earlier: traveling on the road for six weeks at a time. These long periods away from home gave him a good opportunity to survey many of the counties and to meet people over a broad area.

What was left of Martha's nest egg was quickly spent on staples to carry the family through the early part of the winter. Too soon, the cold arrived in Macon County. Fortunately, the boys had learned to be good hunters and there was an abundance of game: deer, wild turkeys, and prairie chickens. For a time, the boys hunted just to bring meat to the table; but as the staples were used up, they hunted to obtain skins to sell. With their earnings they purchased supplies for the family.

Many of the clothes they had brought from Tennessee were either threadbare hand-me-downs or summer clothing that simply was not adequate for the cold winter, so it was necessary for Martha to learn to tan hides and fashion clothing from deerskin. Soon nearly all of her children were wearing pants, jackets, and moccasins made of deerskin. Now they were truly a frontier family.

Abraham continued to be away from home for the usual six-week periods. One time out he made a special trip to Saint Louis to try to get his money back from Rev. Harmon, but the preacher said he would not be able to repay the debt for at least several more months. During the long cold winter of 1836-37, with little food to eat, the Still family had plenty of time to think about the fact that not all preachers were honest, even those who are members of the Methodist Church. However, this was the first time the Still family had a problem like this. (As it turned out, it was several more years before Abraham was repaid; and when he collected the debt, the preacher added no interest for having the use of the money all that time.) The family's second daughter, Mary, was born during that cold winter, adding another mouth to feed.

Martha had always been a good homemaker, but as the winter moved into early spring, she had to take on even more duties. Virgin soil had to be broken up in preparation for planting grain. The family had also acquired a few young pigs and as the pigs grew Martha even learned to butcher hogs. During the evenings, as she repaired clothing and moccasins, she thought a lot about the future of her children. Would the dream of an education for her family ever be fulfilled?

With great determination and courage, a whole lot of help from the children, and only occasional help from her husband, Martha saw her family through this first winter in Missouri. When spring brought garden vegetables to the table and the farm's crops had been planted, she knew – she hoped – that the struggle for survival had passed: they had all stayed alive. One evening, when Abraham was home, the entire family spent the time on their knees offering prayers of thanksgiving for their deliverance.

With the arrival of summer, a few new families moved into the area. They all lived close enough together that it was practical to consider formal education for their children. Although the need was apparent, it would take time to find someone qualified to teach children with so many different backgrounds and ages. It would be nearly two years before the children were able to attend a school.

For their first two years in Macon County much of the children's time was spent getting the farm into production, so there were only two months of the year that could be spared for school. Even so, everyone in the family was certainly getting a chance to develop other important skills. Aside from farm work, the boys learned to hew trees, split rails, and build barns. Now they had a chance to hunt game for pleasure rather than just to bring food to the table.

During this period when the boys were skinning animals, young Andrew became deeply interested in the variations in animal anatomical structure. Why were animals constructed in their own peculiar way, he wondered. How did their muscles and joints function? Could one learn something about human anatomy by a careful study of animal structure? As he meticulously dissected more and more animals, his interest in learning from nature kept widening.

About this time the Still family made another move, relocating about fifty miles north in Schuyler County, Missouri for a couple of years so Abraham could spread Methodism farther to the north and west.

It was the fall of 1841 before the children returned to school. In a four-year period their father had served in four different circuits within the Conference structure. Returning to Macon County, the family settled down again and acquired more acreage. Ed, now sixteen, felt he and his brother would soon have farms of their own. Under the guidance of their mother, the children had been properly trained not only to do farm work but to manage a farm as well.

The girls, including Mary who was born in 1836, hadn't been neglected in this kind of education. They learned much from their mother about what a farm wife should know. In addition, all the Still children were getting better schooling as more and more people moved into northern Missouri.

At first, Abraham welcomed this influx of families. There would now be more people to convert to his church. When he was first sent to Missouri, he was aware it had been admitted to the Union as a slave state to meet the provisions of the Missouri Compromise. But he was of the opinion that most of the slave owners lived either on or south of the Missouri River, and he didn't expect to be confronted with the slavery issue in the northern counties. This had been true at first. Most of the new landowners had enough problems just getting their farms into operation so their families could have a decent living, but as people moved into his area and Abraham spread his preaching beyond and into neighboring counties, he came into closer contact with the slavery issue. It really bothered him that some people moving into his circuits were Methodists who had proslavery leanings. He had been so busy preaching and laying the foundations for future churches and congregations that he failed to recognize a change in attitude of many churchgoers and that some were saying that slavery was of divine origin.

Abraham now had many more places to preach as he helped small groups convert unused buildings into temporary churches, but he could not abide so-called religious people who could hold such inhumane an idea as endorsing slavery. He had always preached against the evils of slavery and for a time there had been only occasional objections. Now, with the influx of more proslavery people he was faced with a division of the church. Some totally approved of his stand on slavery, but soon a greater number began objecting to his abolitionist statements.

On his six-week trips he began to cover an even greater portion of northern Missouri. Each time out, he put more fire into his antislavery sermons. At first, he was told politely to tone down his rhetoric, but instead of following this suggestion, he became more militant in his presentations. Soon his sermons were disrupted vocally. Then there were threats of physical violence. Even the church leaders advised him to slow down or stop preaching altogether and let things quiet down.

Abraham felt that since he had been instrumental in expanding Methodism into northern Missouri and had been responsible for the actual building of the churches and congregations, the region was his domain. If he wanted to preach what he felt was right, no one in the church hierarchy was in any position to deny him his rights as he saw them.

The church leaders persisted. They pointed out once again that Missouri was politically a slave state. They insisted he tone down his antislavery statements. Abraham was so incensed by their request that he added even more fire to his sermons, so much so that he was threatened with physical harm. First it was the threat of tar and feathers, and if that didn't work, it would be a bullet. The proslavery element was tired of being referred to as "godless."

This controversy was not limited to Missouri. The Methodist Church was in turmoil all across the country over the issue of slavery. The conflict grew so intense that in 1844 the church split into two separate units and with Missouri's status as a slave state, the dominant church came under the jurisdiction of the Methodist Episcopal Church South. When this became official, Abraham separated himself from the new organization and for the first time in many years he found himself without a church affiliation.

Abraham continued to feel that the area he had pioneered for the Methodist Church was his personal territory and he should be welcome to continue preaching in what he considered were his churches. He was sure that if he took his message to the congregations, the thinking people would help him convert their brothers and sisters to his antislavery position. He would then be free to once more take his message all over northern Missouri.

For the next three years he functioned unofficially under the Iowa Conference of the Methodist Church, still exposing himself to danger as he added more fire to his antislavery sermons. Each time he left home to preach, Martha feared she might never see him alive again; but his charmed existence continued as he delivered antislavery sermons to congregations in the few churches available to him and to the general public on courthouse lawns.

By 1848, the Methodist Church North was founded in Missouri and Abraham Still was appointed presiding elder to the Platte Mission District in the northwest part of the state, farther away from the most militant proslavery activity. Nevertheless, when Abraham preached he continued to go back to the areas where the greatest threat to his life existed. The new leaders of the Methodist Church North soon realized that this proud, stubborn man who had done so much for the church would be killed if something were not done soon. The church leaders, fearful for Abraham's life, knew a decision must be made.

Finally the new Conference reached its decision. This pioneer preacher would have to be removed from Missouri to save his life and they doubted they could get him to leave the territory through persuasion. They had tried getting his friends and other preachers to tell him he was too important to the Church and his family to keep on risking his life. Since he would not stop his strong antislavery sermons, there was only one way to save him: offer him another great challenge.

Thus, in 1850 Abraham finally agreed to go into eastern Kansas to look at a proposed church-operated mission to the Shawnee Indians. This would give him the opportunity to take his fire and passion into a new area once again. He would not only be in charge of the Mission, but as the church grew in this new territory he would be the Presiding Elder in a position to pioneer Methodism once again. This was too big a challenge for Abraham to turn down. To be the presiding elder as well as the first missionary to a territory that would soon become a brand new state, was more than he could refuse.

Meanwhile, the rest of the family was enjoying a productive period. Martha had two more children: Marovia, born in 1843, and Cassandra, born in 1846. This brought a total of four girls and five boys to the Still family. Fortunately, all of them were healthy. The three older boys had moved onto adjacent eighty-acre farms in Macon County and seemed well on their way to setting up successful independent lives. The younger children were able to attend school on a regular basis, with the quality of their education improving each year.

The major problem facing the Stills when the Conference made its offer was the danger to Abraham when he was on his preaching assignments. For eight years Martha had worried about him. He had been exposed to physical violence on several occasions; his cane had been broken and his clothing rent, and he had also received numerous death threats. Then, too, there was the bitterness the family felt toward their local church. In spite of the fact that Abraham had founded it, their local church had joined the Methodist Episcopal Church South. The Stills attended it for a while, but were faced by enough unpleasantness that finally they avoided church altogether, at least for the time being.

Even under these conditions, Martha felt a real sense of shock when she learned they were going to leave what had become their home state to move to yet another undeveloped part of the country, especially now that they had a nice home, a productive farm, their boys were settled, and the younger children were in school. She remembered in vivid detail that first year in Missouri when they had barely escaped starvation: breaking the soil for the new farm, watching the children struggle to get an education, and facing all this with such courage.

SOMEHOW, A MOVE AT THIS TIME of her life appeared to be a test of monumental proportions. For one thing, they would be moving to Kansas, where there were no stores, churches, or schools. For another, they would be living at an Indian mission. They would see only Indians and an occasional trader.

What made all of this even worse for Martha was that these Indians belonged to the same tribe that had massacred so many of her father's family. She knew that the stories she had heard about the brutal murders of her ancestors would be hard for her to blot out, but she also knew that being married to a circuit riding Methodist preacher was not a life for a person of weak character. Having proven herself in the past, Martha knew she was capable of doing it again, in Kansas.

Chapter Two

ALTHOUGH THE STILL FAMILY had made several moves while living in Missouri, the moves had usually been into nearby counties, and the family had always moved as a unit. Now, Martha realized, this next move – relocating into Kansas – would be the first time her family was separated.

Ed, who had married during the spring of 1848, and brothers Jim and Andrew each owned eighty-acre farms and were in the process of building their homes. Barbara Jane had also married and moved to a neighboring farm with her new husband. Younger brothers Thomas and John were looking at land to settle on when they were a bit older.

Andrew had met a slender, pleasant young lady, Mary Margaret Vaughn. When he told his mother that he was planning a marriage early in 1849, she knew that soon all but her very youngest children would be gone from home. Martha was extremely happy, however, that her family would be living close together. For two years, following the announcement of the move they were to make to Kansas, Martha had plenty of time to ponder about the breakup of what she considered an ideal arrangement – she and Abraham and the younger children all living within a few miles of the grown children and their offspring, her grandchildren.

When they finally started the journey to Kansas, the family on the move consisted of Abraham and Martha, their three younger girls – Mary, Marovia, and Cassie (Cassandra)

– and one of the older sons, Andrew, and his wife, Mary Margaret, with their small infant who was less than a year old.

Andrew and his family had not originally planned to make the trip. The decision was made because their farm had been devastated by a hailstorm on July 4, 1851, leaving them with neither crops nor money. The two had even taken on teaching jobs in order to make ends meet.

During the years in Missouri, Andrew had been allowed to make house calls with his father. So, now, he told Mary, Kansas would bring them better luck and he would have a greater opportunity to learn more about medicine as he helped his father, who with no doctors available, would be looking after the health needs of a very large Indian population.

The Stills were moving into an area with no stores, productive farms, or livestock. This meant they would have to take enough provisions to last for at least their first year, so their three wagons were loaded with enough staples and canned goods to meet this need. They also took two cows, three calves, and a dozen chickens.

It was the first long trip for the younger children. With pleasant weather, the journey to Kansas City went smoothly. When they reached Westport Landing, however, and tried to load their wagons onto the ferry, they were caught in a heavy rainstorm. By the time they reached Kansas City they were drenched.

Their first look at Kansas City was less than inspiring. The "city" consisted of a couple of blacksmith shops, a large general store, and a dozen or so widely scattered houses. It was not an impressive sight when combined with muddy streets that were deeply rutted after the downpour. It didn't appear to them to be much of a city compared to Saint Louis, but it was still the most important starting point for families moving west.

Although Independence, Missouri is usually considered the origin of the Santa Fe Trail and Oregon Trail, some trails actually started from Kansas City and other Missouri towns. The first recorded use of the Santa Fe Trail was in 1821 when William Becknell started west from Franklin, Missouri, eighty-five miles east of Kansas City, and made the nine-hundred-mile journey to Santa Fe, New Mexico with a mule train.

While the Stills were engaged in drying and repacking their clothes and picking up supplies in town, they could watch progress that was taking place in the area. Telegraph poles were being set in place so that Kansas City could be connected with the great cities to the east.

Before they resumed their journey, Abraham thought about visiting the Shawnee mission that had been established before the division of the Methodist Church more than twenty years earlier. It was just across the Kansas line and he had known about it since his arrival in Missouri. He really wanted to see how it was operating since he would soon be managing such an Indian mission himself. However, this particular mission (that would later become a landmark) was now under the jurisdiction of the Methodist Episcopal Church South. Because Abraham had such strong convictions against slavery and such an intense dislike for anyone who supported it, he finally decided against visiting that mission.

After the stopover in Kansas City, the family continued its trip to their new home at the Indian mission, about a mile south of Eudora, Kansas, in Douglas County. It was thrilling for the children. They watched miles of tall prairie grass waving in the breeze. There was such a profusion of wildflowers that, long before the trip was completed, the smaller children had picked bouquets to decorate their new home.

The mission house was a two-story log building that proved to be quite comfortable. But the first year at the mission was a lonely one for several reasons. More than half of the family had been left in Missouri, and the mission and their new home were located miles from commonly used roads. So, except for a few traders, the only people the family in Kansas now saw were Indians.

With the provisions they brought from Missouri they had enough food. There was plenty of good land nearby for development, so it wasn't long before the rest of the family had been encouraged to move to Kansas. Ed and his wife were the only exceptions. Before long the family had several hundred acres of grassland under cultivation and by June of 1853, nearly one hundred acres had been planted in corn.

What worried Martha, as it always had, was that her school-age children weren't getting an education, especially not of the quality she wanted for them. Andrew and Mary Margaret were attempting to teach the younger children as well as some of the Indians. But with Andrew traveling with his father to take care of the health needs of the Indians and with Mary Margaret pregnant, neither could teach on a regular basis. There were many days, therefore, that the children's educational needs were not met.

It bothered Martha that her younger daughters – Mary, Marovia, and Cassie – were starting to speak the Shawnee language. For most of the two years they were living at the mission, mothers and daughters were the only ones at home, so it was natural that the girls learned to speak the language of their Indian playmates.

Most of the Indians were friendly and caused little or no problems. With so many young ones to protect, the women were at first bothered when, more than once, a curious Indian man would look in a window, silently open the door, walk into the bedroom, and look over the clothing in the closet. But then he would leave without saying a word or touching anything.

Fortunately, during their stay at the mission they had only one bad experience. An Indian who had a reputation for being mean when he was drunk tried to break down the door when Martha was away. The little girls were terrified; but before the intruder could gain entrance he became sleepy and was soon stretched out on the front step in a drunken stupor.

During the family's last year at the mission, a terrible outbreak of cholera struck the Indians and because they had practically no immunity to this disease they were dying by the hundreds. Abraham, with sons Andrew and Jim, did everything possible to save them, using all the medicines available as well as Indian remedies made from roots and barks. But nothing had any effect. After such a failure to alter the course of the disease, Andrew pondered not only the cause of cholera, but what could be done in the future to help prevent such devastating epidemics.

There were so many new Indian graves that, after obtaining the Indian chief's permission, Andrew dug up many of the corpses so he could further his knowledge of anatomy. Normally it would have been difficult or even impossible to get permission from the Indians to violate their sacred burial grounds. However, the Shawnees had been relocated several times from their forest homeland to the flat plains of Kansas and in the process they seemed to have lost their reverence for the burial sites. They may also have been so shocked by the great number of deaths and the violent nature of the disease that they were willing to distance themselves from the victims in any way possible.

For a time, Andrew dug up dozens of the epidemic's victims. He was impressed that the muscular contractions resulting from the disease had been so severe. Many bodies were twisted so completely out of their normal shape that hip joints were sometimes pulled completely out of their sockets. With this distortion of the corpses, it had been impossible for the

Indians to bury their dead in any position resembling a normal one.

By carefully dissecting the exhumed bodies, Andrew had the opportunity to do serious study of human subjects. Until this time, he had learned much of his anatomy from animal dissections. During these fresh studies he was deeply impressed with the spine and the nerves that originate from nearly every segment. He wondered about their function.

He was also fascinated by the junction of the last lumbar vertebra with the keystone-shaped sacrum as it sits between the hip bones. Upon dissection, this looked like a very unstable joint. Was it any wonder that so many people complained of pain in this area after an injury or heavy lifting?

For more than two years, he felt free to dig up the graves and, as he facetiously stated later, he never had any complaints from those Indians. But as more settlers moved into eastern Kansas, he considered it wise to curtail this activity. By this time he already had quite a collection of human bones, enough to assemble several complete skeletons.

Perhaps the church had started this Indian mission in Kansas only to get Abraham out of Missouri, but now he was in a position to help the Methodist Episcopal Church North become the dominant Methodist Church in Kansas. The mission was operated for just over three years. Much of its financing had come from a United States government grant to Abraham to provide medical services to the great number of Shawnees who had settled in the area. The mission board of the church didn't have enough money to continue the project, so when Andrew's three-year grant was not renewed the new Conference was forced to close the mission.

After financial support was terminated, the family looked for a new place to live in Douglas County. Abraham found a place on Coal Creek near the Blue Mound area and staked out a claim. Although the boys also staked out claims for themselves, they first helped build the family home and lived in it for the next two years.

The Conference appointed Abraham as the presiding elder for Douglas County. He was urged not only to continue his work as a circuit rider, but to spread his efforts outside the county in order to establish as many new congregations as possible.

One of the high points of his new assignment came when he was asked to help in the organizational meeting that would create the first Methodist Church of Topeka in March 1855. It was a great feeling for him, the Reverend Abraham T. Still, to spread Methodism into eastern Kansas and know that his efforts would not be hampered by restrictions from church leaders with proslavery inclinations.

DURING THEIR YEARS AT THE MISSION, the family had been isolated from the proslavery element that had been the cause of their move from Missouri. But with the move to Blue Mound, and with Abraham's work taking him over a large portion of eastern and central Kansas, he again preached his antislavery sermons, and this again placed his life in danger.

Up until this time, only Abraham had been the target of the proslavery element; but now his children felt as strongly as their father in their hatred of the proslavery views and philosophy being spread throughout Kansas Territory. The children were vocal – as vocal as Abraham – in their opposition.

Martha had worried about her husband when they lived in Missouri. Now she worried about the safety of her children as well. She knew they were definitely a marked family because of this strong antislavery stand.

In 1854 the government made a treaty to purchase land from the Indians. Although the land was not officially open to homesteading until the next year, squatters arrived a year early, sent specifically to promote the proslavery cause. At the same time, abolitionists from as far away as New England joined the movement to prevent Kansas from becoming a slave state. The abolitionists not only raised money but advertised in eastern papers that virgin land was available in this new territory. Many people who moved west in response to these advertisements received some financial support. Those so supported were indoctrinated with a great distaste of slavery on a moral basis as well as opposition to what they called the "plantation economy." These newcomers were sure they would be living in a hostile environment if Kansas became a slave state.

With the influx of people from the South, as well as the Northeast and North, and each group having been sent to see that their sponsors' mandates were carried out, the stage was set for a most turbulent period in the history of this country.

ALTHOUGH THE STILL FAMILY wanted to add to its acreage and build additional homes, all were caught up in the beginnings of action that would soon lead to violence. For a while, raids from Missouri proslavery units were aimed at intimidating farmers who had recently moved to Kansas. In the beginning, such raids didn't cause extensive destruction of property or injuries to the people. But this lasted only a short time as a lawless element, impossible to control, joined the more restrained leaders. Soon farm houses were burned and some farmers were murdered. And the label of "Border Ruffian" was also soon to strike fear in the law-abiding citizens of eastern Kansas.

All families in the Blue Mound area, neighbors of the Stills, shared the antislavery philosophy. As raids by Missouri Border Ruffians increased in number and brutality, and with Abraham, Andrew, and Jim often away on their medical rounds, it was up to the younger brothers, Thomas and John, to see that their mother, their sisters, and brother Andrew's wife and infants were not harmed.

The young Stills joined men and boys from the other families in forming a protective organization, calling it the "Poker Moonshiners" and meeting once a week to drill and discuss ways to protect their families. Along with the Still boys, members included the Ogdons, Landons, Saunders, Smiths, Hougues, Abbotts, and Vaughns. They decided that if they heard that a group of Border Ruffians was in their area, they would meet at the Vaughn house, which was the largest in the area, a two-story structure situated on a hill with a good view. The Poker Moonshiners felt it could be well defended.

On one beautiful night when the moon was nearly full, word spread that Border Ruffians were headed toward the Blue Mound area. John and Thomas rounded up their mother, sisters, and Andrew's family and headed through the woods to the Vaughn house. The family walked silently through the moonlit woods, trying to keep Andrew's two little children quiet. Each time they stepped on a twig or limb, they were afraid the sound would be heard by those bloodthirsty ruffians and they would all be killed. They finally made it safely to the shelter and bedded down for the rest of the night, with some of the men posted outside on guard duty until dawn.

Just as the sun rose, a group of nearly thirty armed men were seen starting up the hill toward the house. After the first fright, they were recognized as members of an antislavery protective organization on their way to Lawrence to meet with leaders and members of a new abolitionist military force. Mrs. Vaughn invited them in to join the others for breakfast.

She needed more meat to serve all these men and went outside to the smokehouse to get some. As she did, she saw about fifteen ruffians heading up the hill toward her.

"Is your husband home, old lady?" one asked.

"Yes. I'll get him for you," she responded, going towards the house.

At this point, the thirty members of the protective force and a dozen moonshiners poured out of the house, their Sharps rifles flashing in the sunlight. The Border Ruffians were so terrified by this outpouring of armed men that they fled in all directions. Fortunately for the residents of the Blue Mound area, the ruffians must have passed on their story about the fortified Vaughn farmhouse, because for a time Border Ruffians didn't come close to the Blue Mound community.

Early in 1855, five of John Brown's sons arrived in Kansas. Near the end of October, John Brown, his son-in-law, and another son arrived in Douglas County. Although Brown stayed in the county for only a short time, the Stills became well acquainted with this antislavery crusader. His ardor and single-mindedness of purpose in destroying all proponents of slavery were a revelation to them. He pointed out that "the sin of slavery must be abolished at all costs."

The Kansas-Nebraska Act was passed in 1854 and set the stage for a struggle in Kansas. The southern states needed to secure Kansas as a slave state in order to maintain a balance between the free states and slave states. It was assumed that Nebraska would join the Free State column.

John Brown was so opposed to any extension of slavery that he felt Kansas should be the battleground where the southern forces would be stopped. And since Kansas was already populated by many people opposed to slavery, this seemed truly the ideal place for him to launch a counteroffensive.

After listening to Brown's fiery and militant speech, people began to wonder if there could possibly be a peaceful settlement of the issue. Brown soon moved his base of operations to Osawatomie, about fifty miles to the south. By this time, Thomas and John Still had become good friends of Brown's sons, particularly Fred.

John Brown, after seeing the need for a strong military unit for the free states, helped induce Jim Lane to come to

Douglas County with the quasi-military company he commanded in Iowa and take command of the established antislavery protective force stationed near Lawrence.

For a brief period, ruffians limited raids into Kansas to an area just a few miles across the border. Since this was a period of little action in Douglas County, and farmers no longer had to spend time defending lives and property, there was an opportunity to start new farms and construct new buildings.

During 1856 the Still family moved from Blue Mound to Palmyra and Abraham and the boys staked claim to a section of land. At the same time, Abraham continued his busy routine of preaching and founding new churches. He was excited when he heard that the Methodist Conference North was planning to establish a new church-sponsored college. This would give residents of this rapidly expanding area an opportunity to obtain a higher education for the first time.

Abraham offered some of his Blue Mound land for the site of this proposed college, but when Conference leaders heard that the state might start a university in Lawrence, the church decided to move theirs farther away. They called a meeting that Abraham, Thomas, and twenty-four others attended, where it was decided that Palmyra, soon to be renamed Baldwin, would be the site for the institution that would become the first university in Kansas. At the same meeting, Abraham made a motion that the new school should be named Baker University after their bishop. This was unanimously approved and again the Stills – Abraham, Andrew, and Thomas – made land available for the college. This time it was 460 acres of their land in Palmyra, representing a major portion of what was to be a 640-acre campus.

This was indeed a busy time for Andrew Still. With the rapid growth of this community and the building of the college, there was a desperate need for lumber. So he and Thomas obtained a steam engine and, along with two other men, started a sawmill. Meanwhile, Andrew continued to practice medicine. He was also involved in obtaining land for the family to replace the property he had turned over to Baker University.

Jim Lane had now organized his military unit, adding many volunteers. They were trained not only to protect eastern Kansas from Border Ruffians, but to retaliate in kind. Following some of the more brutal raids from Missouri when Border Ruffians wantonly murdered entire families, Lane's troops crossed the border. When they caught up with the retreating ruffians, Lane's well-armed forces shot down as many of the raiders as possible. Unfortunately, some innocent people were killed by random gunfire on these retaliatory raids, thus increasing bitterness among many Missourians against the Jayhawkers.

Brown had moved his family to Osawatomie and decided to assemble a military unit under his command to protect antislavery families in the area. There were so many raids and so many abolitionists being killed that he appealed to the courts to have some of the murderers tried for their actions. He was unable to get federal help and no one at the county level would accept any accountability. Failing to get the requested help, he said he would have to take the law into his own hands.

Although John Brown repeated his intentions in speeches and sermons, it is doubtful many people took him seriously. Yet he specifically stated that if these murderous attacks were not ended by lawful means, he would set up his own court of law, put these men on trial, and if the suspects were found guilty, they would be executed. People thought this proclamation was just the raving of a militant old zealot. But John Brown captured five men he considered the worst offenders; after a brief trial by his self-appointed court, he had all five executed by the sword on May 24, 1856. He referred to this as the Pottawatomie Execution. But his enemies called it a massacre.

While the Still family lived in the Blue Mound area, it was involved in a good deal of action and danger. At one time Thomas was captured by a band of proslavery supporters. If one of the leaders had not been befriended several years earlier by his father, the Reverend Abraham Still, Thomas might have met the same fate as others who were captured and never heard from again.

On several occasions when Andrew made his medical rounds he was surrounded by armed proslavery bands, avowed enemies of the free states. They might have harmed him if he hadn't been the doctor attending some of their wives. As it was, he was sternly warned that he had better change his ways, "or else!"

Abraham was on the road a great deal of the time, looking after the sick and preaching strong antislavery sermons, which placed him in constant danger. Since he eluded the danger, it must be assumed that he had a guardian angel protecting him.

It was John Still who was the first in the family to devote himself full-time to the antislavery movement. He volunteered to serve under Lane as a courier, along with several other young men including his friend, Fred Brown. The couriers were to keep the communication lines open between Lane in Lawrence and John Brown in Osawatomie; their duties included carrying the mail and messages as well as delivering supplies and ammunition.

After the Pottawatomie Execution, proslavery units made life even more dangerous for John Brown and his family and supporters. On one of the trips that John Still and Fred Brown made as couriers they were starting back to Lawrence shortly after delivering messages and supplies. With daylight fading, they decided to spend the night in a deserted cabin. The following morning, John began to prepare breakfast while Fred went outside to saddle the horses. A group of men rode up on horseback. When Fred started walking towards them, thinking they were friends, several shots were fired at close range. Fred fell, mortally wounded. On hearing the shots, John rushed out of the cabin to help his friend. When he saw that he could be of no help to Fred, and knowing his own life was in danger, John leapt onto the one saddled horse and took off at full gallop. Although many shots were fired at his fleeing figure, he was uninjured and soon out of range. As he rode on to Lawrence, he was saddened that his report to Jim Lane would be news of Fred's death.

The men who had killed Fred Brown were an advance party of a company of proslavery troops under the command of General John Reid, whose mission was to teach the abolitionists a lesson and, if possible, capture John Brown.

Word of his son's death came to John Brown as he also learned of the advance of a large force of trained military men under the command of General Reid. Brown's first inclination was to protect the town, but when he learned the size of the enemy force and that its ammunition included a cannon, he gathered his men along a riverbank where they would be well hidden by trees. This group, with Brown's sons and a few other men who had been with him for some time, were joined by about thirty-five villagers who supported the free state cause.

As they started to cross the river en route to Osawatomie, General Reid's forces were surprised by John Brown and his men. A fierce battle ensued. It is possible that Brown's unit would have repelled the invaders, but his men ran out of ammunition. He actually lost only three men in the skirmish, but dozens of General Reid's force were killed or wounded. John Brown was able to escape, but seven of his men were captured and about forty houses were burned to the ground.

Up until Fred Brown was murdered and the town of Osawatomie destroyed, many people, including quite a few free staters, reviled Brown's tactics. They were not overly enthused about Jim Lane, either. They felt he was an outsider and a self-appointed military leader, acting moreover as a political leader. Most of the Republicans didn't object, but that certainly wasn't true of the Democrats who called him an opportunist, an interloper, and worse.

The need for good military leadership was apparent after Osawatomie was burned and a subsequent raid on Lawrence resulted in the burning of part of that town as well, so most of the free staters threw their support behind Jim Lane. They told him to form a strong military unit to protect not only their lives and property but their voting rights as well.

The antislavery citizens of Kansas knew that in the days to come, if they didn't have protection, they might not be allowed to vote. That would definitely guarantee that Kansas would become a state in the proslavery camp.

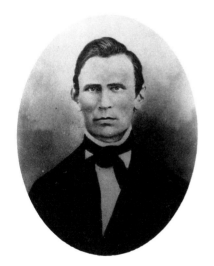 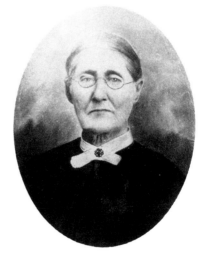

Abraham Still   Mary Poage Moore Still

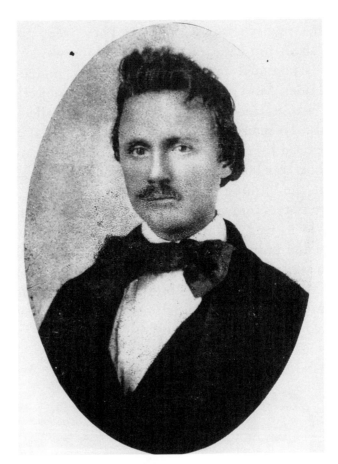

A. T. Still, c. 1850

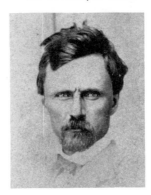

A. T. Still, c. 1860, from a tintype

Chapter Three

NDREW WAS SO CAUGHT UP by his desire for Kansas to enter the Union in the Free State column that he decided to become a candidate for Douglas County Representative in the Territorial Legislature. He was well known in the Blue Mound area and around Baldwin (formerly Palmyra), but he felt it was necessary to meet people from all over the county to get elected. His opponent in the election was from Lawrence and claimed to be a moderate who would not actively support either the abolitionist or proslavery factions or their causes.

As Andrew traveled throughout the county, he was surprised to learn that after all the atrocities committed by Border Ruffians against residents of eastern Kansas, many people blamed the antislavery element – as represented by John Brown and Jim Lane and aggressive abolitionists – nearly as much as they blamed the proslavery cause. Although most reviled Border Ruffians and their raids and were opposed to slavery, they were afraid that if extremists on both sides of the issue continued their warlike actions the country would be torn asunder. With few exceptions, they feared that this warlike activity might spread out of Kansas and Missouri and involve other states in the turbulence that so characterized the border area.

Andrew had felt for some time that a shooting war would come – and soon. As he rode his mule through the county, he discovered most people he met felt that if the extremists would restrict their activities, somehow a middle ground could be found and war could be avoided. Even those with proslavery leanings didn't want the Union they loved to be destroyed. They, too, hoped things would settle down and a peaceful solution found.

Many people in eastern Kansas were new arrivals. To an extent, the newcomers reflected the attitude of those who lived in the middle part of the country. Andrew soon found that to be elected he would have to tone down his antislavery statements. Instead, he must convince voters it would be better to elect a man with strong antislavery convictions – who could best represent the majority of Douglas County residents who were opposed to slavery – rather than select a man who would not commit himself. Many times Andrew had a hard time keeping his strong feelings under control, but in order to be elected and help vote Kansas into the Free State column, he knew he had to stress only the point that he should be the majority's representative.

Andrew Still was elected to the Kansas Territorial Legislature in 1857. He began planning meetings with Free State representatives from adjacent counties – men like John Speer, George Ditzler, and Hiram Appleman. At these meetings, the topic of discussion centered on ways to guarantee that Kansas would become a free state. In addition, Andrew – who had lived in Missouri for twenty years – wanted to be sure revenue from state land would be used only for educational purposes. He noted that some money in Missouri that should have gone into the educational fund had been siphoned off and used instead to help slave owners recover their runaway slaves.

During the county election process slavery supporters realized a majority of counties were probably dominated by antislavery sentiments. As a result, these supporters decided to install a bogus government that would be controlled by men who weren't duly elected. Many of these bogus "Kansas Legislators" were actually Missouri residents who had moved into Kansas. Besides its political power, this element also had military support and intended to make certain that Kansas would become a slave state before the duly elected government had a chance to vote on the issue.

When the counties finally had an opportunity to freely elect their own representatives, an organizational meeting was called. It became apparent that the majority of this new legislature was antislavery and that a truly representative election on the issue of slavery could be held. The date and location for this important meeting were set and Andrew, in a hurry to represent his county and the antislavery cause, arrived about an hour before the appointed time. He was recognized as a free stater by the proslavery contingent and questioned about his political stand. He readily admitted he was there to see that Kansas enter the Union in the free state column. After some heated discussion, followed by threats upon his life, he was reassured to note that other free state representatives were arriving and that they were guarded by several hundred of Jim Lane's troops.

Some free state supporters who had not announced their positions earlier told Andrew he was fortunate to have escaped physical harm and that he might have been a little foolish in taking such a strong political stand in the face of all those proslavery supporters. Andrew responded in no uncertain terms that it was going to take courage and spunk to advance the free state cause. This would not be accomplished by lying back and keeping one's mouth shut, he added.

That evening, the free staters moved into the auditorium early and occupied seats in the rear of the building. Nearly all were armed with Colt revolvers. For a while they allowed the proslavery men to take over the stand and make their presentations. However, some in the proslavery element soon became abusive. There was much name-calling and when one of their more vocal proponents called the free staters a bunch of "sons of female dogs," he was stopped by several hundred free staters rising to their feet with their revolvers drawn. They demanded in no uncertain terms that the speaker be removed from the building. The proslavery men, realizing how strongly they were outnumbered, quickly obliged by removing the speaker and filing out of the auditorium soon after.

By the next morning, there was little or no opposition, so the free staters were able to form their own organization that wholly reflected the ideas, programs, and philosophy of the antislavery majority of the Territory of Kansas. The free staters knew they had won a political victory and that never again would there be organized political opposition within Kansas from slave-staters. But they also knew there would be considerable bitterness as long as Border Ruffians kept raiding Kansas from their bases in Missouri. Such raids were continuing with even greater frequency and intensity.

Another development added to the unsettled situation. There were evil men on both sides of the border. Men from the Kansas side would cross into Missouri and steal slaves, then sell them back to the slave owners. They were called Jayhawkers, a name taken from a mythical bird that raided the nests of other birds. On the Missouri side, equally evil, were men who made raids into Kansas to steal livestock and anything else they could get their hands on. They usually claimed they were part of the politically motivated force that had been trying to intimidate the people of Kansas. As a result, there were retaliatory raids by Jim Lane's troops who chased, and sometimes killed, suspected Border Ruffians and destroyed their bases. These actions originated the claims by Missourians that these men were robbers and murderers, too.

By June 1858, following a two-year absence, John Brown was back in Kansas creating a western extension of the "underground railroad" that had flourished in the east. This operation was intended to free a large number of slaves who would then be helped to find new homes in Canada.

Brown had left Kansas with a price on his head following the Pottawatomie Execution and the burning of Osawatomie. His return exacerbated the warlike state even more. Some people felt that his actions may have been the starting point of all the bloodshed in the territory. As far as the Still family was concerned, however, the drums of war had been rumbling well before John Brown moved into Kansas.

After the excitement of the meeting that created the Kansas Free State position, it was difficult for Andrew to return to Baldwin and get back to his work. However, he was glad to escape the political arena for a while and get his medical practice built up again. There was also the construction of Baker University. It was creating a need for lumber and, although his brother Thomas had been working overtime to meet the needs, the sawmill operation was going to require quite a bit of his time, too.

Andrew hoped he would be able to spend more time with his family, but he seemed to have even less time for it as his practice increased. Mary Margaret hadn't had an easy time while he had been away tending to his political activities. She had never been strong physically, and with her husband away from home so much she had been forced to assume farm duties as well as keep house. In 1855, she had lost a newborn baby, and three months later she was pregnant again. She had high hopes that Andrew would settle down, rebuild a good practice, and either help more on the farm or hire additional help so she could regain her strength.

However, the Border Ruffian raids were still in progress and her husband had strong abolitionist views combined with a love for his country that, she soon discovered, made it hard for him to concentrate on his personal needs – or hers – when the fate of his nation and the antislavery cause were at stake.

Another concern of Andrew's during the time away from his practice was the many failures in the treatment of sick people. He had little or no faith in the medicines that were being used. He hoped that if he discussed these thoughts with other doctors, they might be able to answer some of his questions and relieve some of his misgivings. As a result, he talked to his brother Jim and to several new doctors in the region. Unfortunately, he received little help with his concerns from these professionals. In general, they seemed totally satisfied with the way they were practicing medicine.

Andrew once again returned to his study of applied anatomy. After reviewing the bones and skeletons he so often used when he felt he needed a better understanding of the human body, he began to think that much could be done mechanically to help people with injuries. He began to ponder a series of questions and techniques. Like other doctors, he pulled on or applied traction to a broken limb to reduce a fracture before applying a splint. But what about the low back area in which the spine rests on a keystone-shaped bone that sits between the hip bones? There was often crippling pain in this area that kept injured people away from work and other duties for long periods of time. Couldn't something be done to shorten the recovery time for these rather common injuries?

The usual treatment for low back injuries at that time was to hand out pain pills, and more pills. After reviewing the anatomy of this area, he wondered whether applying gentle manipulation, or maybe even deep pressure, would improve these injuries more rapidly. He remembered that when he was a young boy his headaches were relieved by resting his neck in a swing made of rope or a harness so the pressure was applied specifically to the area where the neck and skull come together. How and why had this procedure benefited his headache pain?

Mary Margaret often watched Andrew in the evening as he pored over his anatomy books and then went to the closet to bring out his bones. At such times he rarely ever spoke, even when the children were loud and knocking things over.

His concentration was so complete that she felt isolated and deserted. They did occasionally have short discussions, mostly about the imminence of war between the North and South. She learned that if a shooting war started Andrew planned to volunteer immediately. Being pregnant again, she wondered if she could endure being left alone once more.

She knew that Andrew was not happy simply following routine medical practice and that he hoped to introduce some of his theories on treatment into his own practice. Actually, he had already started applying his ideas about practical anatomy. He was discovering he could give faster relief to some of his injured patients by carefully correcting minor dislocations and displacements. At the same time, he had reduced his use of drugs without saying much about it to his patients, who continued to do as well as or better than the patients of other doctors.

Finally, he became so disgusted with the general misuse of drugs that be began speaking out against them, particularly against morphine with its addictive qualities and calomel, a mercury chloride compound that often caused major damage to the teeth and gums. This was indeed heresy in the view of the medical profession at this time. The idea that if you were sick you must take something to get well was so deeply ingrained in the minds of the public and the doctors that Andrew's ideas weren't acceptable. Andrew had, however, helped so many patients that his practice continued to grow. His treatments were especially effective for patients who had work-related injuries. In this area he had some spectacular results.

Gradually, as Andrew spoke out against drugs and used hand manipulation with injured patients – a method considered unorthodox – people began to say that he was using some form of "voodoo" medicine. One of the preachers even accused him of trying to emulate Christ by "laying on hands" to cure the sick. As more and more people heard these rumors, his practice dropped off rapidly. Even though he felt his ideas on improving the medical practice were beneficial, he had not yet crystallized them in his own mind. He felt, however, that he had enough answers to be allowed an opportunity to defend himself and his ideas.

Rather than try to answer a lot of questions to a few people at a time, Andrew decided that more could be accomplished if he presented an open forum. Since he, his father, and his brothers had helped in the founding of Baker University and his sister Mary was on its faculty, he asked the president for permission to make his presentation on the Baker campus. The president learned that Andrew wanted to discuss his theories on the use of manipulation in medicine. Being a medical doctor himself, the president decided it would be unwise for such a forum to be held at Baker University, in spite of the university's indebtedness to the Still family. He noted that a college president must often protect his institution from the many "cranks" who would use the campus to present new or strange theories and ideas. Andrew had stated that he planned to condemn the use of drugs and emphasize the value of manipulation. After a brief talk with available board members, Andrew's request was denied.

Mary Margaret shared in the disappointment. Andrew was indeed bitter about this refusal. He knew he had something that was of real value; yet the university he had done so much for in getting it started wouldn't give him a chance. Though Mary Margaret wanted to cheer him up, she lacked the physical strength to do much for him. Andrew was aware that her repeated pregnancies, emotional trauma, multitude of household duties, and the many moves the family had made had weakened her substantially. The emotional impact of people's condemnation of his ideas, added to the recent loss of her child, deepened her feelings of despair.

IN THIS TIME OF WEAKNESS, she often reflected upon her life with Andrew. She worried that her health was failing and was concerned about what would happen to her husband and children if she died. Looking back on her marriage to Andrew at the early age of sixteen, she realized she had repeatedly been in physical situations that nearly exceeded her strength to carry on. During their first year together they had struggled to get their farm into production. It had taken nearly all their strength to plant that first corn crop in their eighty acres of undeveloped land. And she had even had to help Andrew finish building their house.

Shortly after their marriage, she had become pregnant and had been sick and weak during most of her pregnancy. There had been so much to do that it was not until the third year that they got the full eighty acres planted. On the morning of July 4, 1851, they looked over their fields and could see that their hard work should produce a bumper crop. By mid-afternoon, the sky had darkened and, without warning, large hailstones completely wiped out their lovely field of corn. Though neighboring farms suffered some damage, it was Andrew's crop that was totally destroyed.

Continuing her retrospection, Mary Margaret knew that everything was in complete disarray following that fateful Fourth of July just when she had begun to feel secure. A good crop was expected, her daughter was a year old and healthy, and she was feeling stronger. Her strongest feelings of security in those early years of marriage were inspired by the fact that her parents lived less than three miles away. When she had been blue, a short visit with her mother would help dispel her discouragements. Now, without money or crops to sell, she and Andrew applied for teaching jobs to carry them through the winter. She knew that Andrew's parents were moving to Kansas in 1852 and he dreaded their leaving. On the occasions he had gone on house calls with his father, he had found the practice of medicine of great interest and at that time thought he should make medicine his life's work.

Mary Margaret and Andrew had not planned on moving to Kansas with his parents, but the reverses in their fortune caused Andrew to change his mind and they made the move that completely changed Mary Margaret's life. She was uprooted from her parents and friends. After the move, she and Andrew no longer had their own home and were living with her in-laws. At the Indian mission it was a rarity to see white people with the exception of a few traders.

In addition, after the move to Kansas she found she had been assigned to teach Andrew's younger sisters and a number of Indian children. Her husband had intended to help her, but the opportunity to work with his father in ministering to a large Indian population kept him away from home. After the disastrous cholera epidemic, when he wasn't making house calls with his father he had been digging up Indian corpses to dissect to further his knowledge of anatomy.

Still reminiscing, Mary Margaret recalled the last several years in Kansas, how they had moved four times, and how she had had three more pregnancies, losing two infants.

HOW PLEASANT IT WAS NOW to have their own home in Baldwin and how proud she was of Andrew's recent successes in business, politics, and medicine. She believed her religious faith had supported her through some of the rough periods of her life. Here in Baldwin she had found a church home she truly felt would help her through future problems and she often went to her preacher and asked him to pray with her for the safety of her family, not only from the Missouri raiders, but in case her husband had to go to war.

She had been aware that some local people considered Andrew some kind of "crank," but she never thought for a moment that any of her close friends would share such preposterous notions. So she was in a state of complete shock when, one Sunday, their preacher condemned Andrew for his "laying on of hands and trying to emulate Jesus Christ." He further stated that Andrew should be read out of the church membership. And then the preacher proceeded to do so. Although this preacher probably did not have the authority to do this, it had the effect he desired.

Andrew received this proclamation from the pulpit mostly with disgust. He wondered how any preacher could display so much ignorance. But for Mary Margaret it was pure heartbreak. She returned home and for a long time refused to go out in public. Her fifth pregnancy was particularly difficult. After a long and tiring labor, Lorenzo was born. He lived only six days.

For the next seven weeks Mary Margaret tried to regain her strength; although her faith remained strong, her frail body was no longer capable of maintaining life. On September 29, 1859, the thread of life was severed. She was buried beside Lorenzo and another son who had lived only a couple of days.

FOR MONTHS ANDREW HAD WATCHED his wife's gradual deterioration. He now realized that with so many things on his mind he may not have been aware of the extent to which her health had been affected by the recent adversities. He had known how frail she was and hoped to get help for her with the children and house so she could regain her strength. But after she lost her church and her most recent child, she became so discouraged and depressed that her spirit seemed completely broken.

Whatever he had done to help her seemed to be of little or no value. For the last month of her life he had encouraged her to eat enough to regain some strength, but this effort was met with total failure. Andrew had faced many serious physical problems successfully, but in encountering a broken spirit he became completely frustrated. He realized, too late, that he had been so engrossed in his own problems that he hadn't given his beloved wife the support she so needed in time to save her. This experience left an indelible impression on Andrew of the relationship between physical health and health of the spirit.

As he tried to determine what to do next, he realized that Mary Margaret had been a very good wife. She had shared with him some sorrow and misfortune, some successes and pleasures during her brief stay on earth. She left Andrew with a heavy load to carry. Since they had recently adopted a four-year-old girl, he was left with four children – this child (family records do not indicate what name was given to her); Marusha, age ten; Abram, seven; and Susan, six. He had a house, farm, and medical practice as well.

Facing the reality of Mary Margaret's death and the immediate needs of his family, he thought briefly about having his mother help. But he decided that it had been so pleasant for his children when they lived alone as a complete family that somehow he was going to make it on his own with the help of his three oldest children. There would be times, he knew, when he would be away from home for several days at a time and he worried for his children's safety.

Chapter Four

EVEN THOUGH **K**ANSAS was in the Free State camp politically, raids and burning of eastern Kansas communities continued. Even Lawrence, the stronghold of free staters, had been attacked. William Clark Quantrill was feared as the new and brutal leader of the raiders from Missouri. Quantrill made it his business to kill not only men, but women and children as well.

Andrew Still, fiercely loyal to the abolitionist cause, realized that a shooting war was inevitable and he must make preparations to join antislavery troops as soon as war broke out. But following the death of Mary Margaret, he knew there would be difficulties if he went into "the battle for freedom." Nevertheless, he was determined that he must join. He hated to think about leaving the children with his parents, who were already busy. His mother, with her efficient and disciplined ways, was rarely able to show the love the young ones needed, and his father was still away from home some of the time.

While thinking of his options, he met a young schoolmarm from New York state, Mary Elvira Turner, who was living with her sister in the neighboring town of Edgerton. She was in her second year of teaching. After a whirlwind courtship, Andrew convinced Mary Elvira to become his wife. On November 25, 1860, they were married and she joined Andrew and his children on their farm in the Bald-win area.

Although there were still a few raids by Border Ruffians, proslavery forces realized the people of Kansas had spoken with their popular vote in October 1857. If and when the

Territory became a state, it would join other Free States in the Union. There was much to be done before an acceptable constitution prohibiting slavery could be ratified by the people. For a brief time, the Territorial Legislature was involved in hammering out an acceptable compromise in their new constitution.

Most of the fighting and raids were limited to a small area in southeast Kansas and much of the bitterness created by John Brown had subsided. The result was a lull before strife arrived. Though the drums of war were still muffled, many could sense them growing louder. Even on January 29, 1861, when President James Buchanan signed the bill giving Kansas statehood, the big statehood celebration only confirmed that this progress would not have been possible if southern states had not already seceded from the Union.

The conflict seemed nearer and nearer. When the Civil War finally broke out, many Kansans actually felt relieved because there would be no more raids from Border Ruffians. And they were happy their earlier struggles had brought them statehood. There was optimism that this war would be of short duration and everyone could get back to work without any worries about bushwhackers or armed strife. The turmoil that had gripped their lives for so long, they thought, would soon be terminated.

With the war already raging in the east, Andrew enlisted on September 2 in the Ninth Kansas Cavalry at Fort Leavenworth. This unit was soon sent to Kansas City, Missouri and placed under the command of Jim Lane. It was basically a regiment made up of Kansas men who had been been tested under the warlike conditions that had existed in Kansas Territory since the mid-1850s.

There were many in Missouri who felt that since their state was a slave state they should expel any Union troops. General Sterling Price had commanded a Missouri State Guard unit when war broke out and he took over the command not only of the State Guard but also of a new militia, which he felt would represent the proslavery sentiments of his state. Many of Price's troops were from river towns along the Missouri River and these men hated the Jayhawkers. Shortly after it was organized, the militia successfully attacked the Union garrison at Lexington about thirty miles east of Kansas City. Many of the Union troops escaped and made their way to Kansas City. For a time it was thought that General Price's troops would follow and attack them there. However, Missouri had not yet joined the Confederacy and many of the people in that state had taken a wait and see attitude before committing themselves to one side or the other.

After his victory at Lexington, General Price expected immediate support from Missouri, but he didn't get it. With his supplies running low, Price felt he should take his troops and join Confederate forces in Arkansas and should meet with Confederate generals to gain support for his leadership. When General Price's army retreated south toward Springfield many of his recruits who fought at Lexington deserted and returned to their farms.

Andrew's Kansas regiment followed along toward Springfield about twenty miles behind General Price. Although they saw no real action, they saw heavy equipment that had broken down and a number of abandoned wagons. By the time the Union force reached Springfield it had picked up so many antislavery recruits that it had nearly doubled in size. On November 1, the Ninth Kansas Cavalry moved back to Fort Scott, Kansas and three weeks later was moved to Harrisonville, Missouri for the winter.

Although Andrew had joined the army basically to fight for his antislavery convictions, he had hoped it would be on the battlefield. With his background in medicine, however, he was soon serving in the hospital with the title of Hospital

Steward. Many of the troops from Kansas referred to him as "Doctor" and he continued to serve in that capacity during the winter of 1861-1862.

Shortly after the first of the year, Andrew's new wife, Mary Elvira, joined him and served as a hospital matron. Since she was the daughter of a doctor and the wife of a doctor, she was a most useful member of the hospital staff. In spite of taking care of the victims of bushwhackers and the usual number of winter infections, much of the couple's time was spent just waiting. There were many times when they felt they could be doing a lot more at home looking after the children and their farm.

Although the troops stationed in Harrisonville were in no danger of attack by Rebel forces, there were still many men who had been members of the Border Ruffians now acting as bushwhackers and they shot at Federal troops whenever they wandered away from camp in small groups.

Finally, the problem of the bushwhackers became so serious, having caused injuries and deaths, that the commanding officer ordered Colonel Ford to take his Colorado Cavalry Brigade into action. In an eleven-day sweep of the counties, from the Osage River to Kansas City, the Cavalry Brigade reported it had killed several hundred bushwhackers. For the next few months there were no more soldiers ambushed near Harrisonville.

Even after Missouri officially joined the Confederacy, the state remained fragmented in its allegiances. Some areas had strong proslavery convictions; other sections held just as strongly to antislavery positions.

General Price felt that, because the state was committed to the cause of the South and his Missouri State Guard troops had won such an outstanding victory at Lexington, the pockets of opposition would evaporate and Missouri would become a Confederate stronghold. After his decision not to attack Kansas

City and his retreat to Arkansas, General Price had much to ponder. Union troops from Illinois had taken over Saint Louis, and Kansas City was in the hands of General Curtis, supported by Jim Lane and his hated Jayhawkers. With some of his best troops, General Price crossed into Arkansas, vowing that he would soon build a mighty army and return to Missouri as its great liberator.

There was no need to maintain a sizable standing army since there was no Confederate activity in western Missouri. Furthermore, many of the recruits had signed up for only six months. Therefore, it was decided to close several of the camps and send some of the troops home. As a result, on April 1, 1862, Andrew and Mary Elvira and the Third Battalion of the Ninth Kansas Cavalry were free to return to civilian life.

Andrew, like many devoted antislavery men, had joined the army to fight on the battlefield, gain a victory, and return to his home and work. So far, his war experience had consisted of a brief chase after General Price's retreating army. It was not what Andrew had pictured when he enlisted in the army six months earlier. The war in the east was still raging and it now appeared that it was going to be a long conflict. Quantrill was once again terrorizing eastern Kansas with brutal raids.

Andrew and Mary Elvira returned to their home in Baldwin. Andrew's parents had done the best they could with his children, but the children were in need of more love and affection than their grandparents could give them. His farm and home needed much attention and his practice needed a fresh start, yet no end to the war was in sight. Andrew often wondered if life would ever return to a normal state for his family.

Dedicated to earning a victory, he understood that his contribution to the war effort was far from over. He must hold up his responsibility to the cause of freedom, at least until victory was accomplished. Since he so wanted to contribute, on May 15, 1862, he organized a company of militia and was commissioned Captain of the Eighteenth Kansas Volunteers. His company was assigned to patrol the Santa Fe Trail where it passed across Douglas County. It was necessary to drill his unit one day each week, as well as spend additional time on patrol duty.

Soon the unit was enlarged to regimental strength and Andrew was named its Major. The Eighteenth was then combined with other units to become the Twenty-first Kansas Regiment. Its specific duty was to keep the county roads safe for travel, as well as to maintain combat readiness so Quantrill or any other rebel force that might attack Kansas could be repelled.

Major Still soon found that his military duty took a great deal of time away from his practice and the operation of his farm. Nearly two days out of every week were spent in military duty and he often had to postpone his farm work and home repairs. But with Quantrill's raids becoming more intense and daring, it was necessary, for the protection of Douglas County and loved ones, to keep the militia at full strength most of the time. There were few members of the Twenty-first Kansas Regiment who felt that Quantrill would ever attack their part of the state since so many counties were keeping their militia units near full strength. In addition, there were several companies of regular troops stationed north of the Kansas River, just above Lawrence.

"Why would anyone be foolish enough to make more than a few hit-and-run forays into our state?" the reasoning went. Yet Quantrill had been doing exactly that with small bands of ruffians, the largest of which had only sixty men.

It didn't occur to the military leaders of Kansas who made plans to protect the state that they might be vulnerable to an attack by a large force. But Quantrill, having succeeded in his small raids, decided the militia was not prepared to defend against a large, mobile force. Knowing that Lawrence had been the fountainhead of Free State activity, Quantrill targeted that city for one of the most daring raids of the war. On August 21, 1863, he crossed into Kansas with 460 troops and made for Lawrence in a straight line. As soon as Quantrill and his men arrived, they burned Lawrence to the ground. They stole everything of value and killed as many men as they could find before they started their retreat.

The Union troops north of the city thought that Quantrill would follow the shortest route back to Missouri, which was along the course of the Kansas River, so they marched east a few miles before crossing the river and proceeded along the south bank. Quantrill had anticipated this strategy; instead of heading directly to the east, he swung due south in the general direction of Baldwin. With such a quick strike, and with the militia units spread out to protect their counties from small raids, Quantrill felt safe in his selection of an escape route.

The word had just reached Baldwin about the destruction and murders at Lawrence. No one, including Andrew, had thought that Baldwin would be in any danger; that is, until Andrew, repairing his barn roof, saw the fires set by Quantrill's retreating troops. Andrew was not on duty with the Twenty-first at the time since the unit did its patrolling on a split shift.

Many of the Twenty-first were scattered all over the countryside on their usual patrols of the roads. Some were on the eastern border of the county where the Santa Fe Trail came under their jurisdiction. The lack of communication over the distances involved made it impossible to quickly assemble the Twenty-first to full strength.

The fires from the burning houses, barns, and haystacks were drawing closer, and with the possibility that Quantrill's retreating army might destroy Baldwin, too, the first decision made by members of the unit who were at home was to try to protect their families by hiding them in the cornfields.

Andrew hid his wife and four children in the relative safety of their own corn patch. With all wives and children safely hidden, Andrew rounded up forty members of the militia who were not on patrol assignments. With all the guns and ammunition they could find, he picked a spot on a hill where they could wait, obscured by cornstalks that were nearly six feet tall.

It soon became apparent that, while Quantrill was intent on destroying Baldwin, his pursuit by General Lane, Major Plum, and Captain Coleman was too close for him to spend any additional time on the road. So he decided to bypass Baldwin. When Andrew was certain they were not coming to his town, he and other members of his unit told their families good-bye and headed west to join General Lane's pursuing troops. Their late start caused some delay in catching up with the fast-moving Kansas troops. They had hoped to locate Colonel Sandy Lowe, the commanding officer of the Twenty-first, along with other members of their unit, but the others were so far out in hot pursuit of Quantrill that the best they could do was trail along, hoping to see some action if and when they caught up with the rest of the Twenty-first.

Quantrill did an excellent job of confusing his pursuers by suddenly changing direction. In spite of the hot pursuit by many of the Kansas troops, he made it safely back to Missouri with only a few casualties. Except for some of the front runners, most of the Kansas militia units that had joined the chase late decided that they might as well go home. Many hard lessons had been learned. Never again would they leave themselves so vulnerable to an attack by a large force. They must improve both communication and their chain of command.

Although Quantrill never made another large raid into Kansas, he not only accomplished a safe escape but also forced more and more Kansans away from their farms and into using more and more manpower to defend their state from raids. For the next year, the Kansas units spent a great amount of time drilling and patrolling and keeping the militia at full strength to protect against an assault that never came. There were only a few small raids by Border Ruffians.

Many were beginning to feel that continued absence from their farms was a real waste of time and energy. With most of the fighting in the Civil War miles away, they felt they probably would never be needed. The only fighting that had been near them had been during the first few months of the war. It was true that some of the men wanted to see real action, but most would have preferred to return to their normal lives and jobs and not commit all this time to a military assignment.

During August 1864, it was reported that General Price had once more entered Missouri with a large, well-trained army composed of veterans of several major battles, and that he had vowed to capture Saint Louis. Even this seemed a long way from eastern Kansas, but it did send a message that the Kansas units might be needed if Price succeeded. After General Price's forces fought a bloody battle at Pilot Knob, he decided that Saint Louis was too well fortified and he headed west toward Jefferson City.

General Lane called many of the militia officers together and said he felt General Price's real goal was Kansas City, so maybe it would be a good idea to review the readiness of their units in case the Confederate army ventured west of central Missouri and became a threat to Kansas. When it was reported that, instead of attacking Jefferson City, Price's troops had continued west and were spending a few days in Booneville, the Kansas militia was placed on alert. Their commanders were told to bring their equipment to an operable condition to be ready for immediate action.

On October 10, all Kansas units were ordered to report to General Curtis in Kansas City and to get ready to assist the troops stationed there to repel an attack from the Rebel forces. Some of the Kansas units from the western part of the state were not too happy; they had seen no action in the border warfare and questioned whether they should cooperate with this order. But Andrew's unit and others in eastern Kansas were still smarting from Quantrill's raid and their failure to capture him. They were more than ready to report to General Curtis and to be placed under the command of their own General Lane. It was true that many considered General Lane a self-appointed leader, and some disliked his political views, but nearly everyone considered him a good military man.

With the addition of the Kansas militia and General Toten's seasoned troops, General Curtis had assembled an army that totaled well over twenty thousand men. They were waiting along a line that stretched from Independence to the Kansas line. General Price, after leaving the Jefferson City area, moved west along the Missouri River to Booneville. Along the way, he picked up quite a few volunteers. Proslavery residents of Booneville put out the welcome mat. Some of the riffraff who had recently joined his army had no discipline and took advantage of the friendliness of the residents. They helped themselves to horses and supplies of all kinds and rarely paid anything to the people who had so recently welcomed them. General Price was totally opposed to these actions but was unable to enforce his rules on these new recruits.

The character of his army had undergone quite a transformation since it left Arkansas. Some of his better troops had been lost at the battle of Pilot Knob and were replaced by hundreds of these new conscripts who had no training and were totally undisciplined. Another thing that was unsettling to this gentleman/general was the addition of men like Bloody Bill Anderson and Quantrill with his infamous lieutenant, George Todd. These leaders were accepted only because they said they had been retaliating for the atrocities of the Jayhawkers when they raided into Missouri.

With such a heterogeneous and motley army, the Confederates moved quite slowly as they broke camp and headed towards Lexington. General Price realized the danger of such slow movement but was unable to get his troops to move at a faster pace. By the time they were all on the road, Federal troops that had been stationed in Saint Louis started following the slow-moving Confederates.

There were 4,500 seasoned cavalry troops under General Pleasonton, and 9,000 infantry troops under General Smith. Their strategy was to stay close enough to General Price so that when his troops approached General Curtis' army near Kansas City, they would be in position to attack the Confederate army from the rear. The stage was set for what became the largest battle west of the Mississippi River, involving about 45,000 combatants. It was later called the Battle of Westport.

The actual fighting began in Lexington on October 21 and quickly moved toward Independence. For the next two days the battle increased in intensity and by October 24 the Confederate army had moved west, stretching along a six-mile line from Westport south to the Little Blue.

All of the fighting was in Missouri, and some Kansas units refused to cross the state line. They were unsure of their status since they were not federalized troops; they were concerned that they might not be covered in case they were wounded outside of Kansas. They had probably gotten some good advice, as some of the veterans of the Battle of Westport discovered later.

The Twenty-first Kansas was one of several Kansas units that decided it should be part of the action that would help repel the Confederate army and keep General Price's forces out of the state. Several Kansas regiments, under the command of Jim Lane, were brought up to the combat zone and readied for action in case General Price's troops tried to break through the pincher that General Curtis and the federal unit to the east were trying to set up. Major Still's Twenty-first Kansas was in the front line and his men were itching for action.

Andrew was pleased that he was at last going to see real fighting. Many of his troops were still smarting from their failure to capture Quantrill. Andrew, in particular, hoped that he would be a part of the combat and the victory that would insure peace in the West.

On the afternoon of October 24, while protecting the west flank, the Kansas militia units had a chance to show their mettle in a most severe test. They were attacked by Joe Shelby's Iron Brigade, the Confederacy's finest unit. The battle lasted until dark.

Andrew had ridden his mule during the height of the conflict, and although bullets whizzed around him and one even pierced his coat, he was not wounded. But when one of the bullets creased his mule's flank, the mule made such a sudden move that Andrew was thrown violently to the ground, landing on the middle of his back. The mule slipped and rolled over on the lower part of Andrew's body. With the battle still raging around them, Andrew and his mule lay quiet for several minutes, listening to the whine of bullets overhead. Then, when the action moved away, Andrew tried to extricate himself. As he struggled to get his legs free, he felt a sudden and severe pain in his lower abdominal area. He knew that he was injured and possibly had a hernia, but he hoped it was not very serious. He thought that surely there would be more fighting the next day, so it was imperative to get himself and his troops ready.

Joe Selby and many of his brigade had been raised along the Missouri River in the towns of Booneville, Glasgow, and Lexington and had been brought up hating anything or anyone from Kansas. They were deeply disappointed in their failure to rout these unseasoned Kansas militia units. Their disappointment deepened when they were ordered to leave this area and come to the aid of Marmaduke's division, which had been mauled by Pleasonton's cavalry and was in a state of disarray.

When it was learned that the Iron Brigade had moved, General Curtis ordered the Twenty-first Kansas to move to a spot near Shawneetown for the night. The next morning the artillery pieces under General Iotten broke the silence as they shelled the Confederate position. Soon small arms fire could be heard. By noon, much of the fighting had ceased. General Price had ordered a general retreat. With some luck, resulting from poor Federal communication, the Confederate army avoided encirclement.

For the next two days, the Union armies followed General Price's defeated troops. Marmaduke's division no longer existed and many of his soldiers had been captured. Joe Selby's troops protected the rear of what was left of the army that Price had brought up from Arkansas. For all practical purposes, his army had been destroyed. That was not entirely true of Selby's Iron Brigade. As it retreated south, the men still fought some rear guard skirmishes. His defeated troops, still hating Kansas, crossed over the state line and burned houses and barns in their frustration.

Major Still, knowing he had developed a large rupture, was nevertheless back on his mule as his men and other Kansas units followed the Confederate troops in a rout. They passed many wagons and artillery pieces, but mostly they saw sick and wounded enemy soldiers. They felt so much compassion for their former adversaries that they gladly shared food with these men, who in some cases had not eaten for several days.

As the twenty-first approached Fort Scott, Kansas on the night of October 26, it was ordered to encamp there. After breakfast, the men were informed that their services were no longer needed and they could return home. With the exception of a few regular army units, there was no need for manpower to chase the remnants of Price's army back to Arkansas, where it would never again be a factor in the War between the States.

Andrew's days as a soldier had come to an end. There would be no more raids by bushwhackers or Border Ruffians. Bloody Bill Anderson and George Todd had been killed. Quantrill was discredited and had escaped to Texas. There would be no more drilling or patrolling. Word from the east was that the war there was winding down.

Andrew Still could now start his life's work in peace.

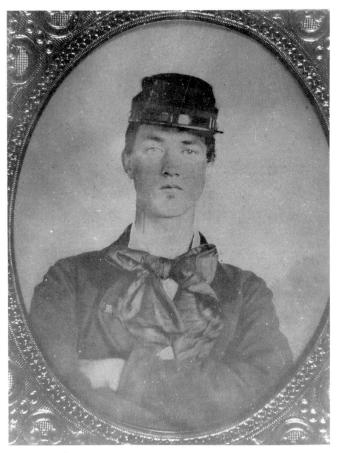

A. T. Still in Civil War Uniform

Chapter Five

HORTLY AFTER HIS RETURN to Baldwin from Fort Scott where the Twenty-first Unit had been released from duty in October 1864, Andrew removed his uniform for the last time. He slumped into a rocking chair and sat for nearly an hour without saying a word. His wife brought him a cup of hot coffee and they sat side by side for quite a while in silence.

When Andrew packed his uniform away, he vowed never to wear it again. He had lost several of his best friends in the Battle of Westport and he was beginning to realize that his own injuries were much more severe than he had at first thought. Some of the other members of his regiment who were either shot or injured in the battle had applied to the state and the Federal Government for financial assistance.

The Federal Government claimed that since the Kansas unit had not been federalized it was not eligible for aid. The state of Kansas pointed out that because the fighting had taken place outside its borders the state was not accountable either. Even though Andrew had not applied for this aid himself, he felt his unit had been treated unfairly in the matter.

Though he was pleased to hear about the success of the Union armies in the east, he was beginning to feel that there wasn't much glamour in war. Truly it was a horrible way to settle even major problems. Not only had he seen death and destruction of property, but now he was seeing something else resulting from the emotional stress of war: a tremendous increase in alcohol consumption and drunkenness. Also, opium and morphine were widely available; with only a few doctors exercising any restraint in prescribing these addictive drugs, another danger loomed.

Andrew was beginning to think that freeing the slaves may have started a trend that, if it were not stopped, would result in another kind of enslavement: drug addiction. This could be as disastrous as the War Between the States, in which so many were now dying.

Mary Elvira had a little boy they named Dudley. He was never too well and lived just a little more than a month. In January of 1863 she had a healthy girl, named Marcia Ione.

Truly 1864 was devastating and a year of great tragedy for them. Even the exhilaration of battle for Andrew had not blotted out the tragedy that occurred that February when a spinal meningitis epidemic struck his children. The writhing of the little ones as he and other doctors tried to save their lives was deeply etched in the memories of Andrew and Mary Elvira. Watching the children's fevers climb and listening to their moans, the doctors realized they were fighting a losing battle.

First Andrew and Mary Elvira saw Susan, age eleven, die; then Abram, who was twelve; and then their nine-year-old adopted daughter slipped away. All died in a three-day period. Fortunately their oldest daughter, fifteen-year-old Marusha, was visiting her grandparents when the epidemic struck and she was spared.

But this terrible February was not yet over; there was more suffering for the couple to face. Following the tragic death of Andrew's children born of his first wife, Mary Margaret, he and Mary Elvira suffered another loss. In the early part of that month, their tiny daughter, Marcia Ione, contracted a chest cold that quickly turned into pneumonia later that month. Although Marcia had always been an active, apparently healthy child, she too died quite suddenly on February 22.

Both parents were devastated again, pushed even deeper into their despair. Had they been so concerned with the earlier deaths of their little ones that they neglected the severity of Marcia Ione's illness?

Andrew turned his thoughts from grief to more immediate problems. Now that he had time to get his farm into production and harvest his crops, he wondered if he had the physical strength to operate it successfully. He knew, however, that his health was good enough for him to practice medicine, but his disillusionment with medical practice made him wonder if he would ever be a good family doctor again. Most of all, he worried about what he could do to help Mary Elvira face an empty house with no children.

But Mary Elvira was pregnant again. Though she seemed to be physically well, she was often discouraged and was concerned about having a family of her own, for now their nest was truly empty. Andrew's one surviving child, Marusha, had become so upset at the deaths of her siblings and with having to learn to live with a stepmother as well that she had decided to stay with her grandparents, Andrew's mother and father, in Centropolis.

In addition, Andrew's two younger brothers, Thomas and John, had decided to try their fortunes in California because of the postwar depression in Kansas. They had been regular visitors to Andrew's home and would surely be missed. His brother Jim was away, also, practicing medicine in Eudora.

Andrew and Mary Elvira really felt the impact of being completely alone now as they faced each other over a dinner table set for two. Immediately following the loss of the children, they had had a lot of company, but now, with all the changes within the family, they were really alone. Only a year before, they had been a complete family with four lively children and a baby; Andrew had enjoyed nearly perfect health, and Mary

Elvira had adjusted to her new married life with this collection of stepchildren, an adopted child, and a daughter of her own.

Even though he missed the companionship of the men in his militia unit, Andrew had great concern for his wife, who could hardly stand being alone, even for a short time, in this now empty house that had been so marked by tragedy. He decided to send her to Edgerton, Kansas so she could be with her sister, Louise Hulett. Louise and her husband had always been so kind, not only to Andrew and his wife but to their children as well. Louise had shared in her sister's loss and welcomed the opportunity to help her with this period of adjustment.

For a brief time Andrew thought about returning to medical school. He heard there was a new one in Kansas City that had replaced the one he once attended. However, his past experience in medical school had been neither pleasant nor very educational. He had been reared as a total abstainer from alcohol and considered drunkenness as a sure ticket to hell, so the regular drinking and carousing of the students detracted from his opportunity to learn. He could only hope that a new school would be an improvement.

A short visit to Kansas City helped him make a decision. The teachers were still stressing empirical medicine with little or no deviation from the text that he had been exposed to earlier. There was no thought of adopting new ideas or concepts. What was just as bad was that there was little or no change in the character or quality of the students or in their behavior.

There was much to be done at home. After checking to see that his wife was doing fairly well, Andrew settled down to the task of getting himself straightened out. The farm work was mostly over for the next few months. Now it was important to set up his priorities.

Andrew had strong feelings about indiscriminate prescribing of syrups and tonics loaded with alcohol and morphine to treat nearly every condition or disease. First, he decided to discuss his concern with other doctors in the area; but his condemnation of addictive preparations fell on deaf ears. For a while, he kept pointing out to the doctors that they must inform their patients of the dangers of the prolonged use of these drugs. The doctors not only didn't pay attention to his concerns, but they joined the public in calling Andrew Still a "crank." Even though he was completely frustrated by the rejection of his warnings, Andrew tried to educate his friends and his patients about these dangers. Only a few, however, took him seriously enough to follow his advice.

This was a particularly troubled time for Andrew as more and more people expressed doubt about his credibility as a doctor. They also pointed out in no uncertain terms that he was hardly qualified to lecture to the public on medical or health matters after he had made such strange pronouncements against the use of medicine. Even worse, from their point of view, was that he believed there were mechanical and structural causes of diseases.

Andrew was beginning to think that maybe the world was not ready to hear new ideas from him. At least, eastern Kansas wasn't. Maybe his ideas were too revolutionary; maybe his theories needed more study and research. Even in his own mind, some of his ideas were only partially developed. They certainly needed more work before they could crystallize into a complete therapeutic system. This might be just the right time to sit back and let his ideas mature. Maybe he should be thinking about something else for a while.

How about some of those inventions he tinkered with from time to time? Often he had helped his wives pound milk into butter when they weren't feeling well. He knew how much of his energy he had used to operate the old dasher-type churn. He realized how much harder it would be for a woman who didn't have his strength. There must be a better way, he thought, to separate the solids from the liquid components of milk. With this concept in mind, he devised a drive wheel, pinion, and rod with attached cups that, when put in motion, would produce butter in less time and with a minimal output of energy. Whenever his new churn was demonstrated, it received immediate approval.

He was soon being told by many housewives how grateful they were for his inventive breakthrough. He was glad to see that so many of his neighbors had constructed his new type of churn and were using the churns in their homes. He was so pleased by the grateful response to his invention that he never once thought about trying to obtain a patent.

Over the years he had watched a mower cut ripened grain only to leave it scattered all over the field. Couldn't a farmer be saved a lot of unnecessary work if some device were developed to hold the cut stalks in some type of container? He reasoned that it would be even better if, after a certain quantity of grain was cut, it was bound into neat bundles of about fifty pounds each so they could be picked up easily without scattering the grain. Using a proper-sized container and long steel fingers operated by a hand lever, Andrew was finally able to demonstrate that bundling the grain could be done successfully. He didn't realize it at the time, but a representative from a large Illinois mowing company was in the audience when he made his presentation. The following summer, while he was thinking about this idea and wondering how to get it patented, he discovered his idea was already in production.

With the acceptance of his inventions by his neighbors, even though he had not received any financial rewards, Andrew and his wife felt they were more a part of the community. Encouraged, he once again thought about making the medical presentation that he had tried to make in the past. Maybe, however, he thought, he should think his concepts through more completely before he made any more proclamations.

On January 1, 1865, Andrew told his wife that with a new baby on the way they must put the past behind them and start all over. A few days later, Charley was born at his grandmother's home in Centropolis. He was such a healthy baby that Andrew and Mary Elvira felt they were on course and it was really going to be a fresh start. Mary Elvira was pleased when Andrew suggested they name the baby after her father, Charles.

Before the spring planting, Andrew had devised a truss he could wear that made it possible for him to do more physical work without bothering his hernia too much. But the spot in the middle of his back was quite troublesome. At times the pain radiated to the front of his chest wall. For a while, he thought he might even be developing a heart problem, since his pulse was so irregular during these episodes.

One day he remembered how he had gotten relief from his headaches by supporting his neck in a swing and applying pressure at the juncture of the cervical spine and skull. He carved a piece of wood so that it was the size and shape of a croquet ball. By lying on his back, with the ball between his shoulder blades, he was able to receive some relief, not only from the back pain but from the radiated constriction in his chest as well.

Many times Andrew wanted to speak out about the inadequacy of medicine as it was being practiced and the injudicious use of drugs by doctors, as well as about his own ideas on manipulative medicine. But he had come to the conclusion, from past experiences, that if he were to build and maintain a practice he should no longer antagonize people. Besides, he realized that he still needed answers, and only by treating patients could he further his research on the relationship between structural changes and disease, if there was such a relationship.

Andrew had always possessed an outstanding ability to correct dislocations and reduce fractures. Could his sensitive fingers, he wondered, help him find structural changes that might be characteristic of certain diseases?

Over the years, he had noticed that nearly each acute infection had its own special qualities, such as different types of rashes or fever patterns. And, as many country doctors claimed, each disease had a characteristic smell. Although Andrew had been well aware of these diagnostic pointers, he was now beginning to find that there were also muscular contractions along the spine that occurred in nearly every acute infection. They, too, followed a rather specific pattern for each disease. Was this the breakthrough that he needed to help him develop a specific system of therapy? He had known for some time that there were loose ends to be tied into a neat package before he could make such a proclamation.

For the present, the most important thing was to see as many patients as possible and give them the best care possible while continuing to see if it was true that there were characteristic reflexes or structural changes present in all diseases. This entailed a study of normal tissue to establish criteria that would make it possible to differentiate the normal from the abnormal.

Andrew never lost sight of his objective to find a better way to meet the needs of his patients, whether they were injured or sick. He knew there must be a better way than forcing dangerous drugs into a sick person, or bleeding an individual who was already weak. He never lost confidence that he would find a way to do this, and he knew that he must now really buckle down to expand his understanding of the mechanical cause of disease.

As his interest increased in giving his patients the best care along with doing research on his own, his practice grew rapidly. He had learned his lesson about making his thoughts known regarding new concepts. He also made no more public statements about the dangers of drugs, except to a few patients who he knew would take his advice.

For the next few years things were really looking up for Andrew and Mary Elvira. Twin boys, Harry and Herman, were born in May of 1867. The couple had added to their farm and acquired enough good help to make theirs one of the best farms in the Baldwin area. Best of all, because of Andrew's ability to be a good doctor they were now one of the most respected families in Douglas County.

There were times, however, when they could not shut out the memories of those fateful years when they lost their first family.

IT HAD BEEN A FEW YEARS EARLIER that his parents moved to a farm in Centropolis where his father, no longer needed as a circuit rider, was still active in the churches and congregations that he had helped found. Abram continued his work of spreading Methodism, even into the central part of Kansas. Whenever he had the opportunity, he was happy to fill in for any preacher who needed him.

On Christmas Day, 1867, he honored a request to fill in for a preacher in one of the churches he had founded. Although he hadn't been too well himself and was seventy-one years old, he got out of a sick bed and preached what was reported to have been an "outstanding sermon." On December 31, he developed an acute attack of pulmonary congestion and died.

Six of Abram's children gathered at the funeral to honor this pioneer circuit rider. They also honored their mother as a pioneer, for she had braved the worst that the frontier could offer and yet had been strong enough in character to see that all of her children acquired an education. What would become even more unusual is that during a period of great infant and child mortality all but one of her children would live into the twentieth century.

When the children told their mother good-bye after the funeral, they felt confident that she could run her home and small farm by herself. There was nothing about Martha Still to suggest that she couldn't.

Shortly after the funeral, Andrew decided to talk to his brother Jim again. Jim had once been his favorite hunting partner and Andrew felt bad that they had drifted apart. Maybe he had been too critical of Jim and the way he practiced medicine. He soon realized that Jim was not going to forgive him for his utterances, and that Jim still held doubts about his sanity. This dispute would continue to color their relationship for many years into the future.

As a parting shot, Andrew told Jim he hoped he would be the first in the medical profession to grasp the truth of the mechanical and structural causes of disease; that he hoped Jim would be the first "pup in the litter" to open his eyes. Later Andrew would use this same expression in a prayer to the medical profession in general; but at that time Jim was not impressed. They each went their own way and didn't cross paths again for several more years.

FOR THE NEXT FOUR YEARS, ANDREW kept the promise he had made to himself. He kept his mouth shut while doing his best to properly administer an ever-growing practice. He had confirmed several of his thoughts about the presence of spinal reflexes in specific diseases. In addition, he discovered there were changes in the temperature of the skin. Sometimes the abdomen would feel cold and the area over the lumbar spine would feel hot. This condition was often found in association with severe diarrhea.

For a while he observed these anatomical changes without doing anything therapeutically. What was the cause of these reflex changes? Without saying anything to the patients or their families, he tried rubbing the involved areas. Then he found that by applying deep pressure he seemed to produce better results. He had also, on occasion, applied heat to the cold areas and cold to the warm spots. His final conclusion was that deep pressure over the area of the reflex, with his skilled hands, was the best way to shorten the course of an acute infection.

He now felt that he had tied up all the loose ends, that he had the breakthrough he needed to complete the work he had started, and he had a totally new system of treatment. He knew that he could keep his ideas to himself no longer. Gradually, he began to tell his patients, then the public, that he had manipulated patients with acute infections and had been able to shorten the course of their disease.

The public accepted his treatment of injured patients. They accepted his use of his hands to reduce dislocations. But when he once again started talking about treating infections by manipulation rather than by the use of medication, the public and even many of his own patients again doubted his sanity.

Financially, the Stills had done well. They had acquired more land and during the spring of 1873 had added to their livestock. Nonetheless, Andrew was still bitter about this most recent rejection of his therapeutic concepts. He knew that he had finally developed a system of treatment that could revolutionize medical practice, if only he could find open-minded people to whom he could explain his concepts and techniques.

Beginning in 1870, and for three years in a row, Kansas farmers experienced weather conditions that were nearly ideal; they were able to raise fine crops, add to their livestock, and even build additions to their homes. Many of the farmers had borrowed to the limit at the banks.

But during the winter of 1872-73 no snow or rain fell and there were no spring rains. The outlook for a good crop that summer disappeared when May and June brought no relief from the drought. Soon with no crops and with many farmers on credit and at the same time needing more money to feed their livestock, the whole state found itself in a deep financial depression. Many banks were closed and many farms were lost. Some families faced starvation.

Andrew and his wife were barely able to maintain even a small part of their farm and lost most of it, as well as most of their livestock. Again, Andrew was deeply discouraged; and once again former patients and his neighbors were questioning his medical skills as well as his sanity.

By that October, with no crops, no money, and little respect, he became quite depressed. Some of his old ailments grew worse and, as winter took hold of eastern Kansas, he developed a deep chest cold that would not go away. He felt so bad that he was unable to do even the lightest, most essential chores. With his wife pregnant again, he felt that it was imperative to make a major change in their lives.

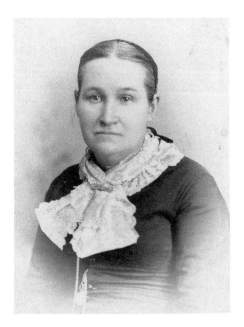

Mary Elvira Turner Still

Chapter Six

HE MORNING OF JANUARY 7 broke cold and clear. Charley Still watched the pale yellow sun try, with little success, to dispel the cold of a winter night in eastern Kansas. He felt chilled to the bone as he proceeded with his morning chores. The horse was given its morning ration of hay and oats, the hogs were slopped, the chickens fed. Last, he milked the one remaining cow. As he picked up the half-filled milk pail and headed for the house, he thought about how the crop failure during the summer of 1873 had been so hard on all the families he knew. He had heard that some families in western Kansas had even starved.

Charley was glad to get into the warm kitchen and join his younger brothers in a breakfast of biscuits and gravy. The twins, Harry and Herman, helped their mother straighten up the kitchen. She was expecting a new baby and it was difficult for her to do her usual household activities.

The boys put on their coats, stocking caps, and mittens, and headed for school, their coat pockets stuffed with the rest of the biscuits. It was a long, cold walk from the Still home to the schoolhouse and they heard the school bell as they rounded a bend about a quarter of a mile away.

"Well, we'll be late again," Herman observed as they increased their pace. During the walk to school, Charley had paid little attention to the complaining of the twins. Harry had repeated the same theme many times: how boys shouldn't have to do women's work. At other times, Charley had pointed out that all of them must do everything to help their mother since their father was sick and another baby was on the way.

Today, however, he felt sorry for himself. It was his ninth birthday and no one had even wished him a happy birthday. He felt a little bit better as he seated himself at his desk, feeling the warmth from the potbellied stove.

Miss Wilson, their teacher, had put her hand on his shoulder as he was removing his coat. Maybe she knew it was his birthday. She had been so nice to the family when she stayed at their home. Like most of the early teachers in Kansas, she didn't make enough money to rent a room of her own, so she boarded around with the families of her students. She would have loved to have a private room where she could have some peace and privacy, but for a while, she knew, she could not afford it. When staying with some of the parents who had little or no education it was hard for her to find much in common with them in the way of conversation or discussion. This was certainly not the case at the Still home. Andrew had taught school and practiced medicine. Mary Elvira had gone to college in New York State and had then taught school in the neighboring town of Edgerton.

The first year of Miss Wilson's stay in the Baldwin area had been highlighted by visits with the Still family. Although all her families were having a hard time, things seemed to be worse at the Still home. Like many who had lost their livestock and even their farms, they were trying to rebuild. Some were doing so with moderate success, but Miss Wilson wasn't so sure about the Stills.

Andrew had a good medical practice and a fine farm, but he seemed to have lost interest in both. Miss Wilson had heard that in the past he had condemned medical practice as it currently existed, had claimed that drugs were of no use, and said that there was a mechanical cause for disease. Now, once again, he was expounding his medical concepts to anyone who would listen.

Miss Wilson had also heard that on moonlit nights he was often seen roaming the countryside. Some people, who knew of his past actions at the Shawnee Indian Mission, claimed he was digging up graves. Being in his room so much during the day and taking those long midnight walks during the summer and early fall stirred up rumors about his sanity. It was not surprising that some of the students greeted the Still boys with, "How's your crazy Pa?" The schoolteacher had punished some students who were taunting the Still boys. She found that Harry, large for his age, never avoided a fight and stopped many younger children from making unkind remarks about his dad with his fists.

While Andrew's patients were leaving him in search of doctors who would provide pills and other medicines, he spent more and more time alone in his room, studying anatomy and concentrating on the human bones in his collection. During this time he let his family look after the house and what remained of the farm. If they hadn't done all the work themselves, the family might have lost everything.

Miss Wilson knew enough about Andrew's dedication to what he called "research" to realize that he truly was a man with such single-mindedness that he just might come up with something of medical value. But she could not help but feel some resentment for the way he treated his family.

This day, Miss Wilson looked out the schoolhouse window and watched the snow begin to fall and the sky turn a leaden gray.

"We'll close early and all of you had better hurry home," she announced. She checked the windows and banked the stove, preparing to leave the schoolhouse. A quick glance at the school calendar reminded her that in about eight weeks her young male students would be absent as they would be out in the fields preparing for spring planting.

Meanwhile, at the Still home, Mary Elvira was frustrated and saddened as she prepared the evening meal. She had been so uncomfortable lately with her new baby on the way that she knew she hadn't fed her family properly. She hoped that soon she would be able to prepare decent meals once again.

"Today I'm going to fix one really good meal for my eldest son's birthday," she said aloud to herself as she began preparing the evening meal. She brought in a few pork chops from the smokehouse and peeled a dozen potatoes for the boys' favorite mashed potatoes and pork chop gravy. Most families have cake for birthdays, but in the Still household Andrew and the boys preferred pie. Each would select the pie of his choice and then Mary Elvira would bake two large pies as part of the celebration.

The wind and snow had increased and the walk home from school had worn out the boys as they battled the cold blowing snow. The twins went right into the house to thaw out, but Charley decided to do his outdoor chores and be sure that the animals were properly prepared for the bitterly cold night.

As soon as Charley entered the house, he knew that his mother had done some baking. Such a wonderful smell filled the air! As he went around the kitchen stove to warm up, he spotted the two pies.

"Are they gooseberry?" he asked.

When his mother nodded, he knew she had not forgotten his birthday, after all. He didn't say anything for a while. He just gave his mother a big hug.

"Is Pa coming down for dinner?" he finally asked.

"No," she replied, "his fever and cough have gotten worse. He's going to stay in bed. He does know it's your birthday, though, and he's sorry he can't join us."

The boys were so tired that shortly after the kitchen was cleaned up and the dishes put away, the twins went to bed without their usual bickering. Charley waited around long enough to thank his mother for the birthday dinner and to give her another big hug.

For the past two nights, Andrew's cough had been so bad that Mary Elvira hadn't been able to get much sleep. Tonight, since Andrew was already asleep, she decided to sleep on the couch downstairs. She knew her new baby would arrive soon and it was necessary for her to get a bit stronger to face the rigors of another childbirth.

She thought to herself, "As sick as Andrew is, will he be able to deliver me this time?" She tried to put the thought out of her mind. He had made her other deliveries so easy for her that she couldn't think of having another doctor for the birth of the new baby.

"I must get a good night's sleep," she kept repeating, and settled down on the couch, trying to properly cover herself against the cold that permeated the room.

She had never slept downstairs before and was surprised at how noisy and drafty the room was with the strong north wind blowing. There were times when the whole house seemed to shudder. In addition, the barn door kept slamming in the wind because Andrew hadn't fixed the latch. He really hadn't repaired anything lately.

She tried to sleep, but found it impossible to keep her eyes closed with so many strange sounds. She pulled the covers up over her head to try to shut out some of the noise and to keep warm. Soon, however, the chill of the room seemed to take over both her body and mind.

Her thoughts raced without control back to her earliest days in Kansas. The little town of Edgerton where she had joined her sister and had taught school had been so unlike the tree-lined streets of Newfield, New York, where she had been raised.

Gradually, coming back to the present, as she lay on the couch she realized that without some heat to dispel the chill she would be unable to get any sleep at all. After checking to see that her husband and children were asleep and well covered, she started a fire in the kitchen stove. Soon the heat from the stove and the coffee she heated made her feel better. As the room warmed up, the movements of her unborn baby increased to the point that she was sure she would be unable to get any sleep. But because she was too tired to sit up any longer, she returned to the couch, blew out the lamp, and pulled up the covers.

LYING IN THE DARK ROOM, listening to the shuddering of their frame house in the strong wind, she again began to reminisce. She thought of those early days in New York state when she and her sister Louise attended college together at the Poughkeepsie Female Seminary, and the pleasant days when she helped her father run their small drugstore.

She had learned a good deal about sicknesses and the compounding of drugs from her father. She had thought many times that if only women could be doctors she would surely have entered that profession. How dramatically things had changed in her life when her mother died rather suddenly. She had still enjoyed working with her father in the drugstore, but living at home with a new stepmother had become a rather unpleasant experience. When her sister Louise married and moved to Kansas, Mary Elvira realized she would soon have to make a major change in her life.

She had felt so alone after Louise left, and, at times, unwelcome in her own home. When a letter from Louise arrived telling her of an opportunity to live with them and teach school in Edgerton, Kansas, it took no time at all for her to make up her mind to head west.

Although her father hated to see her leave, he had been aware of the problems at home as well as of her loneliness. His two daughters had always been inseparable. He wished her the best and in his final admonition, which he repeated twice, said, "Stay close to Louise. I know the two of you can handle any situation."

The trip to Kansas was a lot harder than she could have imagined. She was thoroughly worn out. It was hard to tell which was dirtier, her or her clothing, when she stepped down from the wagon and was greeted by Louise and her husband, Orson Hulett.

The next morning, after a good night's rest, she took a long hard look at her new home and the schoolhouse where she was to teach. What really impressed her was that the small town of Edgerton had no tree-lined streets. In fact, there were hardly any trees anywhere. With little rain during August, there were hardly any lawns or green shrubbery, either. There was really nothing to greet her eyes to make her feel that this would be a good place to live. How different from her former home!

Her biggest shock occurred on her first visit to the schoolhouse. It was a combination of frame and mud walls with a dirt floor, nothing like the well-built school she had attended back home. She was nearly in tears when her brother-in-law, Orson, drove her back to their farmhouse.

She felt a bit ashamed of herself during the next few days, because Louise had done so much to make her feel at home. She concluded that with so much love and attention surrounding her things would work out all right.

Even before school started, Louise began teasing her about coming west to get a husband. But the men Mary Elvira had seen around Edgerton were not the type to inspire romance. They were mostly farmers in overalls and boots, and they had lots of whiskers. Many of them also used great quantities of chewing tobacco.

She had told her sister that if she did find a suitable man there were two things she would not accept in a husband. One thing was his using tobacco. The other thing that would be totally unacceptable, she declared, was if he were a widower and had children.

She had never taught school before and, even with her good education and background, she soon found it a real challenge to teach these children who came mostly from farm families. The medical training she had obtained at her father's drugstore came in mighty handy for treating the many minor injuries and illnesses that she felt well qualified to treat.

She found she liked to teach, and she liked the children. Even though she missed her former pleasant surroundings, she felt that she could be happy in her new location and that Kansas could truly be her home from now on.

Her first year as a teacher moved along at a rapid pace. She proved to herself that she was a good teacher and capable of taking care of her students' health problems. However, during the following spring there was an epidemic of scarlet fever in eastern Kansas. Mary Elvira had been able to diagnose it in one of her students and called in one of the local doctors to treat them.

That is how she met Dr. Andrew Still for the first time. He not only confirmed her diagnosis, but seemed pleased to meet a young woman who had such a good education and a good background for treating the common ailments found in a rural school.

As other students contracted the disease, Andrew made more and more visits to Edgerton and always spent quite a bit of time visiting with Mary Elvira. He was a tall, handsome man who had a kindness and gentleness in handling sick patients.

It didn't take her long to find out that he not only chewed tobacco, but he was a widower with three children of his own plus an adopted daughter. She learned that his wife had been dead little over a year, his youngest child was six years old, the oldest daughter was ten.

Andrew had really struggled trying to keep his farm and medical practice going. There were house calls that took him away from home for hours at a time. Trying to find help to look after the children and the house hadn't been too successful. He really felt that his children needed more love and affection, and if Mary Elvira would consent to be his wife, he was sure his children would have someone special who could give them the care, love, and attention they so sorely needed.

Besides, Andrew not only admired this young, educated schoolteacher, but he began to feel that he was truly in love with her. Even though he needed her to help with his family, he would have wanted her to be his wife simply because of the way he felt about her.

As for Mary Elvira, she had felt she was falling in love with Andrew from their first meeting. His sense of humor when he was with her, the constant twinkle in his eyes, and his ability to create a feeling of confidence in his patients, all really appealed to her. Since there had been times when she had wanted to be a doctor, she felt that if she couldn't attain this ambition for herself, perhaps being married to a doctor would give her a firsthand opportunity to be involved in medical practice, if only as a helpmate, for she knew how to compound drugs and knew a lot about illness.

Even without all this, she found herself hopelessly in love with Andrew and so, after he promised to give up chewing tobacco, she promised to marry him. She hated to give up teaching. Most of all, she would miss the evening talks that she and Louise had shared almost daily.

Although her love made her minimize some of the problems she felt marriage might create for her, she was still hardly prepared for the sudden and drastic changes that occurred when she moved to Andrew's farmhouse twelve miles from her sister Louise. She had thought, however, that she was mentally prepared for her new role. She had met other challenges before without too much trouble. She also felt capable of being a good wife and a good mother to Andrew's children. However, there were other responsibilities she hadn't considered. For one thing, she had never kept house for a whole family before. She had helped her sister, but feeding and cleaning up after her new husband and his four children took a lot more time and energy than she could have imagined was possible.

Then, with Andrew gone from home so much of the time as he made house calls and ran the sawmill, she found she was also expected to see that the farm animals were fed, the cows milked, and do all the other chores that were daily requirements for operating a farm. There were times during those first few months of her marriage that she wondered whether she was capable of handling all her new responsibilities. But whenever things got too rough, she would load up the wagon and drive the twelve miles to visit her sister Louise. Living near Louise proved to be a lifesaver during this time. Sometimes, when Mary Elvira was the most deeply discouraged, Louise would bring some of her children over for a surprise visit. It seemed that Louise was able to anticipate when she was most needed.

These visits gave Mary Elvira a chance to really let down her hair and to find that her sister also had experienced some of the same problems. Louise was also able to offer some solutions that had helped Mary Elvira adjust to married life.

The disruption caused by the war and the tragedy of the disease that struck down Andrew's children made Mary Elvira even more dependent upon Louise. So – even after her own boys were born – she continued her regular visits to the Hulett farm. It was hard to be away from Andrew, but she felt her boys enjoyed meeting other children who were unaware of the things kids in Baldwin were saying about their father.

Knowing that her sister was near enough for regular visits made it easier for Mary Elvira to face the most difficult situations, but these visits were tenuous because of Andrew's intense concentration on his new theories in the field of medicine. Things weren't being taken care of when she was away visiting. Andrew often forgot to feed the farm animals and it finally became necessary to find someone to help him with the chores.

The Huletts had made several additions to their farm over the past few years. They now had a sorghum mill and a large apple press, so twice a year their farm became a center of activity. Even though this entailed a lot of work, these occasions were festive celebrations. Shortly after the sugar cane was harvested, many of the neighboring families would load their cane into wagons and head for the Hulett farm. Besides the cane, they also loaded in all their children and lots of food for a picnic lunch.

While the juice was being squeezed from the cane and transported through a long pipe to the sorghum mill where it was cooked to the desired consistency, the families spent their time visiting. The children played and the food disappeared. Then the sorghum was properly divided and loaded onto the wagons, and the families headed back to their own farms. The sweet smell of sorghum hung around the Hulett farm far into the night.

Even as pleasant as the sorghum operation was, it didn't compare with the fall apple festival. There was a lot of work involved in processing the apples into cider and vinegar. Nonetheless, this two-day procedure always took on a festive air. There was more time for the children to play, even more food to eat, and more time for visiting. This was a major celebration for the Still children and a chance for Mary Elvira and Louise to do some real visiting, with their discussions often lasting far past midnight.

The first day of the fall apple festival began when the apple-laden wagons arrived from the nearby farms. Soon the men were busy feeding apples into the press powered by a horse hitched to a long pole. As the horse walked around and around in a big circle, gallons of apple juice were produced. Soon there was enough apple juice to furnish each family with a year's supply of cider and vinegar. After filling all the jars, bottles, and jugs, the families loaded their wagons and headed for home.

The second day of the 1873 fall apple festival was most enjoyable for the children. As the men were busy unloading the apples and the women were kept busy peeling the fruit, the kids could play all sorts of games without interference from their parents. Some of the women set up the picnic lunch, but most were involved in peeling and cutting the apples into small pieces, which they put into a large copper kettle. With a wooden paddle nearly as large as an oar they kept stirring the kettle of apples vigorously to prevent scorching.

The women took turns stirring. While this was going on, a long and, at times, rather loud discussion would take place about what spices should be used and how much of each should be added to produce the perfect apple butter. The apples were almost always sweet enough, so no sugar was really needed. On that point the women could nearly always agree. But while a few women were still arguing over the spices and the amounts to be added, the apple butter process went on to completion. Jars were filled with fragrant, tasty apple butter, again enough for a year's supply for each family.

The festival ending, the wagons were loaded, the children stopped their play, and the women and men cleaned up after the operation. Soon they all headed towards their own homes.

During most of the second day of the festival, as the sisters watched their children play, they had serious discussions. This time talk was about the changes in Andrew and the effect this was having on his family. Louise noted once again that their own father had certainly been right when he told them, "As long as you two stay close, you can handle any situation."

BRINGING HERSELF BACK TO THE PRESENT, Mary Elvira noted that the wind was gradually dying down, the creaking and rattling sound that kept her awake had abated, and for the first time during that long night she finally slept, her mind at rest in deep sleep.

Upstairs Andrew awoke, racked by one chill after another. His chest was painfully constricted but he was unable to cough. He also felt that if he didn't move soon, he would be unable to breathe at all. He nearly fell as he moved over and lit the lamp. Then suddenly he felt something loosen up in his chest. He grabbed a basin and, without warning, he brought up copious quantities of dark, prune-colored sputum. He noticed that he was bathed in perspiration. Being a doctor, he knew that his fever had broken and that he should change into a clean nightgown.

Back in bed, he began thinking once again about what had been on his mind lately, something he was going to have to tell his wife. For some time he realized it would be necessary for him to make a major move. He knew he would never again be accepted in Douglas County. Too many people here were critical of his neglect of both farm and family. In addition, few would ever come to him as a doctor after he had so boldly announced his ideas about the proper way to treat sick patients. His new concepts were still considered sheer lunacy by the other doctors in the area and most of the general public also shared their opinion.

When his family had first moved to Kansas and lived on the Indian mission for the Shawnees at Eudora, he had felt free to dig up the Indian graves to further his knowledge of anatomy. And he had had the permission of the Shawnees to do that. Although there were very few people in Kansas at that time, there were still some living there who remembered his early digging. They called it "grave robbing." Local rumors persisted in Baldwin that he was involved in what the people considered ghoulish activities. Of course, as the population had increased at Eudora, he had given up collecting bones. Now he realized there was nothing he could say or do that would change the ideas of many of these people. If he were to develop a good medical practice once again, one in which he could experiment and add to his new concepts, he knew he would have to move a long way from Baldwin.

For a long time he had thought about making a move, but it was just recently that he finally made the decision to return to Macon County, Missouri, where he could practice with his brother Ed. He knew his brother hadn't been too well lately and would probably welcome some help.

He felt the move wouldn't be too hard on the boys, but for his wife it would mean leaving her sister, Louise, and that might be devastating for her. But he knew it had to be done and that he must tell her right away. He had tried for several weeks to get up his courage; although he had faced many kinds of difficulties in life without backing down, this situation would require added strength.

Suddenly, he thought of his mother and how she had left her pleasant home in Tennessee, and with her five children and her circuit riding preacher husband had moved to a mostly unpopulated area in northern Missouri. She had assumed the duties and responsibilities of a frontier wife, and that had taken real courage.

Andrew could see a light burning downstairs and knew his wife was awake. He felt a bit shaky as he walked down the steps, but he knew this was the time to tell her of his decision.

"Mary, I feel better. My fever's gone," he said. He always called her Mary, for he disliked the "Mary Elvira" that her sister and others called her.

"Mary," he repeated, "there is something I have to tell you. I think you had better sit down. I have decided to return to Missouri to practice with my brother. I know I can build a good practice once again if I get away from here."

Mary was speechless. For a moment, all she could think about was how hard it would be to leave Louise. Then her thoughts shifted to Andrew. As shocked as she was by his pronouncement, she was relieved that his fever had broken. He had been so sick that in the past few days she had worried not only that he wouldn't have the strength to help her deliver their baby, but that his own life might be in serious danger.

Although Andrew had known for some time he was going to leave Kansas, telling his wife that he had decided to move to Macon was one of the most difficult things he had ever done. Now that he had finally found the courage to tell her – now that he had accomplished this – he felt much better.

No longer worried about telling Mary Elvira of their pending move, he enjoyed better health and was able, by the twenty-fifth of that month, to deliver their fourth son, Fred. Andrew was thrilled. He felt he was ready, once again, to get back into his special field of medicine.

"Maybe," Mary Elvira thought, "after we move to Missouri and Andrew establishes his medical practice there, he will again be the dedicated, kindly man who had so attracted me when we first met."

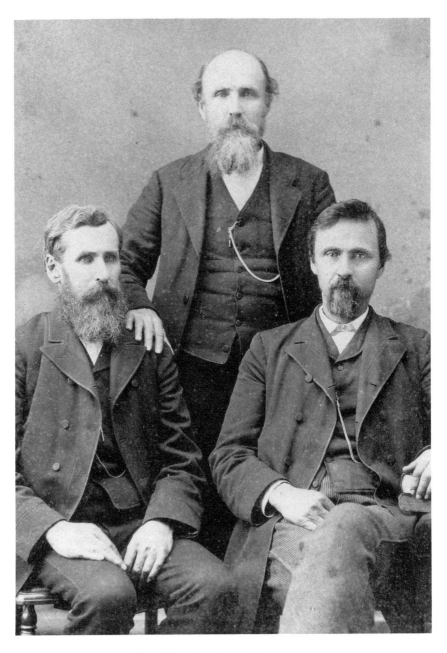

A. T. Still and his brothers Thomas and Edward

Chapter Seven

NDREW AND MARY had had their conversation and he had told her of his decision to move to Macon. Now that he was feeling better, the two could sit down and discuss their plans together. He was slowly getting his strength back from his long illness and he planned that as soon as the weather warmed up he would travel to Macon to make preliminary arrangements for the move back to Missouri – at least for himself, for he was going in advance of the family.

He remembered Missouri hadn't been too kind to him in the past and there were still bitter memories of how the first crop on his first farm had been wiped out by a hailstorm and how he and his first wife had nearly starved and had to ask his parents for help. He also remembered how fortunate it was that his father, so outspoken against the proslavery movement, had not been killed by that element in northern Missouri. And how his father and mother and the rest of the family had been driven out of the church that his father had founded by the intolerance of other church members. Finally, he remembered how it had been necessary for the family to move away to protect his father's life.

In addition, there were his memories of the Border Ruffians and the troops who had fought in the Battle of Westport. Still he had committed himself to return to Missouri and it was necessary for him to make the best of this move and do his utmost to forget the past. There was so much to do, that there certainly was no time for him to be dwelling on the past.

During the previous year he had made several trips to Macon. When he and his wife began discussing plans for the move, they decided they could wait awhile before taking the final steps. There were still things to be done on the farm. He was feeling better and it was important to get the farmhouse and barn in the best possible shape so they could sell the farm. Mary Elvira was rapidly regaining her strength from childbirth and Fred, the new baby, was sleeping so much she could help her husband as he painted and fixed up the house and the farm buildings.

Except for a vegetable garden, they decided not to do any planting that year. Andrew would have to move by late spring and the boys were too young to think about operating a farm. He felt that now he should take time away from the hours usually devoted to his daily study of the human body and development of his new science and instead enjoy his wife and children before moving to Macon ahead of his family. Most of his skeletons and anatomy books were already packed and ready for shipment.

Mary Elvira hoped the change in scenery would bring the family closer together and for the first time was feeling better about their move to Missouri. She told Andrew that after everything on the farm was fixed up she would concentrate on raising garden vegetables and doing as much canning as possible before the move.

Andrew thought it wouldn't take too long to get his practice going in Macon so that he could rent a house and send for his family. It was almost the first week of April before things were in good enough shape for him to leave his family.

This trip was intended as a short one to find a place to stay and to visit with his brother. He found that Ed's health had deteriorated during the winter. Ed had been taking several drugs and when Andrew examined him, he found Ed was dependent upon an addictive drug. Unfortunately, as Ed's health worsened, many of his patients left his practice. Andrew discovered that his brother wasn't going to be so helpful, after all, in starting a practice in Macon. Nevertheless, the die had been cast and it appeared that it would be up to him to build a practice on his own. First, though, he must help get his brother back to better health.

Andrew made a couple more trips back home to Baldwin. Near the end of the third week in June 1874, Andrew unpacked his belongings – clothes, medical supplies, and everything else he would need until the rest of his family arrived. He put all his possessions into the single room he had rented in Macon and realized at this point that he had cut ties with Kansas.

He had crossed his Rubicon. He had committed himself to a definite decision, final and irrevocable. So on the twenty-second of June, 1874, he announced the discovery of his new science. But as yet it didn't have a name. He would later say that he flung the banners of "Osteopathy" to the breeze on that date. Whether or not there was anyone present to help him celebrate this occasion was never recorded. It was true, however, that at the time his proclamation was made it apparently had very little impact on either the medical profession or the residents of Kansas and Missouri.

While the world would, many years later, record this date as the beginning of Osteopathy, at the time there were no announcements in the newspapers nor was there anyone in Macon with whom Andrew could share this moment. There was only his brother, who was too sick to be involved.

The year 1874 received little attention in Missouri history. However, it was notable in Kansas, where it is remembered as the year of the grasshopper. Billions of the winged insects descended on the state that summer, totally destroying crops and leaving the water supply contaminated with their decaying bodies.

Although Andrew had been quietly practicing drugless manipulative medicine almost exclusively for several years, he felt that his complete break from Kansas was the real starting point of his science. He could now proclaim that he had developed a complete system of treatment, a wholly different school of medicine. Even though he had made the proclamation of his new profession, it still didn't have a name. So for the time being, in the eyes of the local people he would be considered just another doctor.

After setting up a small office in downtown Macon, he took time to meet some of his brother's former patients. He was a bit surprised when he found that Ed had said so little about having a brother from Kansas who was coming to help him and his practice, or that this same brother was planning to stay and make Macon his home. For a while, Andrew thought this oversight was due in part to the drugs Ed was taking, which might have affected his memory. But as Ed's health improved and he was able to walk around town, he obviously was still reticent to recommend his brother "Drew" to his patients and fellow townspeople. This became so obvious that, one day, Andrew confronted Ed and asked him point-blank what the trouble was. His brother finally dug out a letter from their brother Jim in Eudora, Kansas. Jim wrote that anyone who took on Drew as an associate would be in real trouble, that Drew had surely lost his mind, and that his crazy ideas about medical practice would certainly ruin not only a practice, but make him a target of ridicule from the townspeople. Ed told Andrew that he had not shared these views of Jim's with anyone else and he agreed not to do so in the future.

Now that he knew why he had gotten so little support from Ed, Andrew realized it would take longer to get a practice started than he had first thought. It would also take longer before he could send for his family. It was time to buckle down so that this time, when he got his practice established, it would be his exclusively. It had also taken longer than he expected to get registered in the county as a physician and surgeon. Finally, on August 29, 1874, he was notified that he was duly certified to practice in Macon County.

His first few patients were those who had sustained some kind of joint injury. He had met some of them in the post office and at the courthouse. A few came to his office for treatment, but many were treated wherever he found them. Often, he just used the wall of the handiest building to support them while he made a correction. Since most of the cases were injury related, it didn't seem too strange to the patients that he used no drugs. He had actually seen so few patients during his first months that there were not too many people in town who paid any attention to this new doctor.

This changed rather suddenly. A severe epidemic of acute diarrhea struck the town, the kind that caused a high mortality rate, especially among young children. As a result, it was referred to as "bloody flux." In the past, Andrew had good results treating simple cases of diarrhea by manipulation. Although he hadn't treated cases like these before, he offered his services to some of the poorer families. After several spectacular cures, he was called on to see many more seriously ill children, and his results continued to be outstanding.

It was not until the epidemic was over and he had gotten his results without the use of medication that the people began to talk about the strange powers that allowed Dr. Andrew Still to drive away the demons of sickness through some magical use of his hands.

Before Andrew had a chance to enjoy his success, however, the local Methodist preacher heard about his miraculous cures and how they had been accomplished by the "laying on of hands." He took the pulpit one Sunday morning and declared that this new doctor in town must be possessed by some unnatural spirit and could become a dangerous element in the community. The night before his sermon, the preacher had met with Edward and told him that he considered his brother a most dangerous person and he felt it was his duty to rid Macon of his evil influence.

After the preacher's sermon, many people crossed to the other side of the street when they saw Andrew approach. The preacher's statements from the pulpit, followed by additional gossip, created so much fear in the general population that Andrew soon saw his dream of moving his family to Macon and making this community his new home fade away completely.

He did continue to try to practice in Macon for some time. Since he couldn't go back to Kansas, at least for a while he had no other option. He was faced with another losing battle and he hated to have his wife and children subjected to even more ridicule than they had received in Baldwin. He must do something; but what? He thought about it upon rising each morning. He dreaded to walk the streets, seeing people who considered him dangerous and, possibly, some type of strange creature.

The decision to leave Macon was indeed a bitter one for Andrew. He had just gone through one move, and he hated to think about another one. But the hardest part was the letdown feeling he experienced. He had come to Macon with so much enthusiasm for a fresh start and the hope that he could soon send for his family. In addition, he knew that it would be shocking news for Mary Elvira when he told her about his change in plans and the delay in having the family join him. Besides that, he missed them so.

As he finally finished his packing, he wondered why the Macon preacher had made such an effort to drive him out, especially since he had really benefited so many who were ill during the epidemic. He asked Ed if he had discussed any of his problems in the Baldwin area with the preacher. Ed reminded him that he had promised to keep that information to himself and he had done so. Ed seemed as puzzled as Andrew about why the preacher had started his vendetta against him.

Andrew had visited in Kirksville, a little over thirty miles from Macon, and had also met a few of its citizens. They seemed friendly on his visit. He had to do something soon. Mary Elvira had sold the farm back in Kansas, which after the grasshopper scourge, hadn't brought them much. They were being allowed to stay on the old homestead for another six months; then they would have to move. He knew that his family could stay with the Huletts for a while, if necessary, but he was faced with the decision that he himself must move and he had to find a new home for his family soon.

It was not difficult for him to decide on Kirksville. He knew it was a bit too close to Macon and that rumors would probably catch up with him. However, several of the people to whom he talked seemed open-minded, as well as friendly. He met a lady named Mrs. Ivie, who ran a rooming and boarding house, and she told him that he could stay with her for the first two months and pay later. It took him very little time, after his decision was made, to gather his possessions and put them on a train for what proved to be his last move, this time to the town of Kirksville, Missouri.

His wife had a little money from the sale of the farm. She was selling magazines, so she was able to send him a small amount of money to tide him over until she could join him. Naturally, she had to keep something to finance her move, so it was a very lean time for Dr. Still.

One of the medical doctors in town, a Dr. Grove, who was a bit of a maverick himself, took a liking to the doctor who had successfully treated so many sick children and then been run out of Macon. Dr. Grove took it upon himself to encourage Andrew to start a practice in Kirksville. He introduced Andrew to a man named Charley Chinn who had a small office building, and between the two of them they convinced

Andrew to rent a small office in which to set up his practice. Once again, he was allowed to pay later.

Dr. Grove had heard of Andrew's skill at reducing dislocations, so he steered a few patients in his direction. Charley Chinn, who knew how discouraged this new doctor must be, came regularly to Andrew's office to cheer him up. He was always repeating a saying, "One day, you will outride the storm."

With the support of Dr. Grove, Mr. Chinn, and a few other townspeople, Andrew's small practice began to grow. It was a very slow process, but it was a start. By late May of 1875 he felt it would be all right to send for his family.

With all their money gone, Andrew and Mary Elvira knew they had a high and steep hill to climb. Although they had already experienced some tragic times, the two were now facing one of the most difficult periods of their lives together. It would take a total family effort, but they were all together and all healthy. And they had found new friends in a new hometown.

Andrew's practice was bringing in such a small amount of money that they were financially strapped, and the unpleasantness of his brief stay in Macon on top of the last couple of years in Baldwin made it doubly hard for Andrew to get the mental strength and heart to face all the complexities of starting over.

When she left Kansas, Mary Elvira had left the sister who had always given her encouragement and friends who had helped her build up a fairly good business selling magazines. She, too, would have to start from scratch to supplement the family income. There were many evenings after the children were in bed that she and Andrew wondered if it would be possible to outride the storms of adversity that surrounded them.

They seemed to have reached their lowest point when one day ten-year-old Charley came home to announce that all by himself he had gotten a job in the local printing office as a printer's devil, which meant he was an apprentice to the printer. He was so proud of his accomplishment. Mary Elvira and Andrew were pleased and their spirits were lifted to the point where they knew that as a family they were going to surmount whatever obstacles might lie ahead.

Soon the whole family was involved in helping. Harry and Herman, the twins, were doing odd jobs, and Charley was working regularly after school. Mary Elvira was once again selling magazines, and Andrew's spirits were raised again. It took nearly six months before they could start paying back their debts; nonetheless, they knew that they had gotten over a major hurdle and that things would be better soon.

The battle, however, was only partially won. There were many local people who considered Andrew a "crank." Kirksville was so close to Macon that there were people who would ride the train to repeat the remarks and accusations that their preacher had made. In spite of this, Andrew's practice now rested on a firm footing and he was slowly earning enough so that it was a lot easier to pay the bills.

He still had quite a bit of free time, and he felt fortunate to have met a gentleman by the name of Robert Harris. This man had spent most of his life as a gunsmith and machinist. It was a pleasure for Andrew to have someone who had such a good knowledge and understanding of mechanical principles to talk with. They spent many hours discussing how mechanical forces and principles could be used to understand the functioning of the body, especially the actions of the joints and muscles. These hours of discussion helped Andrew later in explaining to patients his theories of human mechanics and their ramifications.

To increase his practice, Andrew made numerous house calls to patients out in the country, sometimes as far as six miles from home. Many times these calls to the more remote farmhouses would take him where there were no roads and he often had to walk through muddy fields and climb fences.

Later on, when the boys were a bit older, he would often take one of them with him on his jaunts to the country to help serve the sick. He always took his bag of bones along so he could demonstrate what he was planning to do. Often, when he was headed for the country, he would call out to the nearest son, "Bring the bag of bones. We've got sick people to see."

Competing with the local doctors was a real problem in the beginning. Being such a nonconformist, Andrew refused to dress like the other doctors in the community. Some of them wore tall silk hats and other items of formal attire. Andrew's rumpled suit, slouch hat, and worn boots didn't give him a very professional appearance. His habit of sticking his pants into his boots in a most inelegant manner added to his bizarre appearance.

One of the other problems he had in competing with the local doctors was that he would not use the title "M. D." But, as yet, he had no name for his type of therapy. He also never attempted to be a part of the medical community, even if the other doctors would have accepted him, which was doubtful.

Not having a name to describe his services, he had on occasion advertised as a "magnetic healer," even though he thoroughly disliked its connotations. He had spoken of himself at times as a "human engineer," but that didn't cover the scope of his services either. There were men in other parts of the country who had exceptional skill reducing joint problems. They were referred to as "lightning bonesetters." He didn't like this descriptive term either, but because of his ability to reduce dislocations he was soon being called that by some of the public.

Even with some outstanding local successes and a few people who had faith in him, there were still many people who feared deviating from the orthodox system of treatment. These people made it difficult for him to build much of a practice in Kirksville. Besides the farm families who lived near the town, there were many other small towns near Kirksville that had no doctor. For a period of time, Andrew decided he would join the ranks of itinerant doctors who visited these communities. He had handbills printed and distributed announcing his arrival in their community upon a certain date and time. He also advertised that if they had any joint problems he would be glad to see that they were corrected.

He had such an ability to select cases that would benefit from his services that before long he had built quite a reputation in those communities surrounding Kirksville. He often treated patients in front of twenty to forty people. After a demonstration of his skill, he would give people an opportunity to ask questions about what he was doing and what he might be capable of doing.

These demonstrations and appearances sharpened his skills as a lecturer. He learned to stay away from medical terms and speak in a language that nearly everyone could understand. He also stayed away from the medical "hocus-pocus" that so many of the itinerant doctors used. He never tried to explain his theories, only the mechanical principles involved in making a joint correction.

His trips to the small communities and the farms around Kirksville gave him plenty of experience, but because so many people were obviously poor, even poorer than his own family, Andrew refused to take pay for his services. So, in spite of being busy most of the time, his financial situation improved at a snail's pace.

All this activity with his remarkable results soon began to bring patients into town. While Kirksville had not quite accepted this strangely attired doctor yet, they were beginning to take notice of him as patients from the surrounding areas arrived in town and asked where Dr. Still had his office.

Since Andrew's trips had brought in so little money and were so tiring, Mary Elvira finally convinced her husband to stay home more. "Let the people come to you," she kept stressing. Andrew hated to give up his trips to the country and small towns. He could see they were such an opportunity to lecture and people seemed impressed by these appearances. Finally, however, he agreed to spend more time in his office in town. In the long run, he probably would end up with more money and he could conserve his strength. Even so, he agreed only to curtail the number of trips, not to end them entirely. That was the best that Mary Elvira could get out of him.

The boys were now attending school and local families were getting a chance to meet other members of the Still family. G. I. Brundage later reported: "I first met Charley. He was about my age and we were schoolmates. Soon we became fast friends. We spent many nights together, at which time I would be close to Dr. Still; sometimes rather closer than I would have liked. He always had a box of bones and skeletons around his study. I remember that I, along with many others, thought that he was a little 'off.' We only knew about doctors who used drugs and my family, like many other families, couldn't figure out what he was trying to accomplish.

"The Still family was in a financial bind at that time, but we knew that even though the 'wolf' was never far from their door, A. T. [Andrew] would buy groceries for some of the poorer families that lived near him, even when he could hardly afford food for his own table."

Other children who played with the Still children heard their parents say that Dr. Still must have some strange power because, according to reports they had heard, he was able to cure people without the use of drugs of any kind. Although by now many people in Kirksville knew about Dr. Still, there were still very few using his services. Some of the ones who did sneaked around so that they would not be seen going into his office.

FINALLY A BIG BREAK CAME. The Reverend J. B. Mitchell, an outstanding Presbyterian minister with one of the largest churches in town, who had a crippled daughter who was unable to walk, came to see Dr. Still at the urging of his wife. However, there was much criticism of Andrew's unorthodox methods; and some of the minister's congregation, who had moved from Macon, considered Andrew possessed by Satan. Rev. Mitchell told his wife it would be unwise to allow such a person in their house. Mrs. Mitchell learned her husband was going to be out of town for a week and after he left she met Andrew on the street and asked him to see her daughter. She also asked him to come in the evening so the neighbors wouldn't see him and report back to Rev. Mitchell that she had disobeyed her husband. Andrew agreed and was able to treat the child twice before her father returned.

After the second treatment, the girl was able to walk down a flight of stairs unaided. From then on, Andrew made his visits in the daytime when he could be seen by any of the neighbors. After a nearly complete recovery, Rev. Mitchell stood with his daughter before his congregation and declared that he had complete faith in Dr. Still's method of treatment. He gave Andrew a vote of complete confidence.

It was quite a twist of fate and seemed paradoxical that while Andrew's father had pioneered Methodism in northern Missouri, Andrew's church support had come from a different denomination. In contrast, his father's church had done so much to make life miserable for him and his family and to destroy his practice and discredit his approach to medicine.

For the first time, local people felt comfortable going to his office any time of day. The big breakthrough had finally arrived. He was now seeing quite a few local patients, along with those from the outlying areas. Mary Elvira and the children were being accepted by the community and, for the first time, their financial difficulties began to fade.

For the next several months things went smoothly for the Still family. Andrew's work was getting a more favorable reception, Mary Elvira was able to meet and get acquainted with some of the ladies in town, and the children were making friends who were not worried about their father and his collection of bones.

It now appeared that Andrew, who had developed his science some time before and had been practicing his special type of therapy for several years, could now concentrate on expanding his concepts even more, without having to worry about earning enough to support his family.

Unfortunately, this was not to be the case. In the period when he was debating whether he should enlarge his office space, Andrew contracted a severe case of typhoid fever. For several months he was in a very serious condition. After surviving the acute phase, the resulting weight loss and exhaustion forced him to spend an additional three months in bed. His recovery from typhoid fever was extremely and painfully slow. When he was finally able to get around, he was a far cry from the strong, robust man who had returned to Missouri in 1874 at the age of forty-six. His hair and beard had turned gray during his sickness, his abdominal muscles had weakened, and once again his hernia was a problem. His walk was unsteady and he needed a staff to support his emaciated body.

When he lived in Kansas, his brothers, sisters, and close friends had called him "Drew," townspeople usually called him "Doc," and his nieces and nephews called him "Uncle Doc." Now, following this sudden aging, nearly everyone who knew him well started calling him the "Old Doctor," but with much affection.

Once more, the Still family was faced with adversity. Andrew's practice was gone and with his health in such an uncertain condition, it was hard to tell whether he would ever be able to rebuild and carry on a full practice again. Mary Elvira and the boys had to seek additional work just to keep the family from total financial collapse. Fortunately, the townspeople, many of whom had by now been treated by the Old Doctor, were quite helpful. They hoped that he would be able to practice again. With his slow recuperation, many were resolved to help the family as much as possible. Nearly everyone admired Mary Elvira and the boys for the "spunk" that they had shown earlier and how they had now taken hold again.

Before he had the strength to walk any distance, Andrew would sit in the backyard and study the animals carefully. He patterned his life-style and some of his ideas about how to lead a healthier life by closely observing their behavior. He had such a deep love of all living creatures that he felt much could be learned by watching how they adapted to their environment and the stresses of their existence. He noticed that a mule, after a hard day's work, would roll around on the ground for several minutes, stretching every muscle, then slowly drink water before it would eat a bite, even though it may not have tasted food for many hours.

From his studies, he came to the conclusion that the birds and animals living the longest never ate too much at any one time and were also more likely to be physically active. He reached an opinion that an overstuffed stomach prevented the free flow of blood to the heart and lungs, with possible dangerous consequences. Even though he had a sweet tooth, he had earlier established moderation in his eating patterns. He felt that meals of many courses and long sitting with lots of conversation were a sure ticket to an early exit from this life. He felt that discipline during the holiday seasons in the consumption of food was essential to a healthy body. Overeating, too much sitting, and too much talk should be eliminated. One of his favorite statements was, "Did you ever see an owl eat and hoot at the same time?"

Andrew had always enjoyed his morning walks, and just as soon as he regained some of his strength he began walking again. He finally worked up to a quarter-mile walk before breakfast. He spent nearly a month with these short walks before he ventured uptown.

His favorite place to visit was Henry's Drug Store. He had several friends who gathered in the drugstore every day and "batted the breeze." The Old Doctor often referred to these sessions as "having the jollies."

Mrs. Henry later said that whenever the Old Doctor had some loose change he would look around the store to find some inexpensive item that a child might like. He'd save his gift until one of the poorer children came into the store. Since many of these children were also dirty, he would pick up a small bar of soap and suggest that the child use the soap, along with accepting the gift. Even before his strength returned he continued to bring friendliness and good cheer to his visits in the drugstore.

Andrew was unable to practice during this period of recuperation, and Mary Elvira finally talked him into writing to the government about his war injury. He had always said that the government didn't owe him anything, but his wife convinced him that perhaps the government did owe something to his family.

His hernia was definitely the result of his war injuries, so finally he applied for help. He knew that some of his army buddies had applied for help not too long after the Battle of

Westport and had been turned down. He hoped that the policies had changed so that the Kansas militia could receive the same consideration as the regular troops.

He wrote requesting that the government consider his case. He reported that he served under the command of General Curtis and that his unit had been asked by the general to cross the state line to help repel the upcoming Rebel attack. Because they had followed the orders of a Union general, he stated, he felt they should receive the same consideration as the regular troops.

After some time, he was notified that the same regulations were in force: his request was denied. When he received this reply from the Bureau of Pensions, Andrew was furious. He had filed his claim on November 20, 1877, and the government had waited five months before responding.

"If they were going to turn me down, why didn't they let me know sooner?" he raged.

What he considered grossly unjust treatment by the country he loved so much just made him resolve to get his anger under control, get out his bag of bones, and once more hit the road to practice. His wife suggested that maybe he had better start in town rather than on the road.

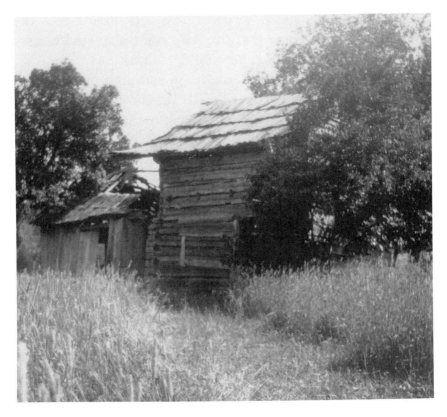

Abraham Still Cabin, *in situ,* Virginia

Chapter Eight

FOR SEVERAL MONTHS, beginning in the spring of 1878, Andrew Still again saw as many local patients as his health would allow. He was affected by the fact that when he had first come to Kirksville he had advertised himself as a "magnetic healer." Not liking that description of his services, he quickly dropped it. He had never become a member of the local medical community nor listed himself as a Medical Doctor. Since he hadn't developed a name for his special services, he was often referred to as a "lightning bone setter."

Once more the urge to spread his services to more people in need, as well as to enjoy the stimulation of visiting smaller towns, led him to spend quite a bit of time on the road. His strength was returning from the recent bout with typhoid fever, and he enjoyed performing in the small towns more than in the the larger communities.

Kathryn Talmadge, a resident of one of the small towns not too far from Kirksville, later wrote in a letter:

> Years ago, when I was a small girl living in Schell City, Missouri, I heard my mother discussing a wonderful doctor she described as a "bonesetter." She had made up her mind to try his treatment, as a last resort, to see if she could get relief from a pain in her right side which had kept her an invalid for years. Our family all held its breath until the "miracle man" came to our town. Meanwhile, the doctor was making trips through different parts of the country demonstrating his new

science, which had not yet been named. We, at that time, did not know this traveler was our beloved Dr. Still.

At last came the eventful day. The town turned out to see what might happen: some from mere curiosity; some in the spirit of those who went to our Savior to be healed. These did not go away disappointed. They found a most kindly man who worked not for pecuniary reward, but for the love of humanity. When my mother told the doctor about the pain in her side, which had baffled all medical skill, he just smiled, pressed on a rib, gave her arm a twist, and assured her she would have no more trouble.

It was hard to believe, but as time passed, we all began to have faith and the pain never returned from that day on.

With so many successes in dozens of small communities, Andrew again contemplated the wisdom of setting up a branch office in some other community. He had looked over several prospective sites and decided that Hannibal, Missouri, the home-town of Mark Twain, might be a good place to have his first office outside of Kirksville. He finally made a decision and established a timetable for making this move. Although he had planned to open his branch office in the spring of 1879, the death of his beloved sister-in-law, Louise Hulett, near Thanks-giving of 1878 caused him to delay his expansion plans for quite some time.

Mary Elvira was so tied down with their children that she was unable to go to Kansas to help the Huletts. Although it took Andrew several weeks to get things in order so he could be away from home for a while, he managed to go to Edgerton, Kansas, to assist the surviving Orson Hulett and his children. Andrew was reassured to find the family making a brave effort to carry on. Mary Elvira, deeply saddened, was thankful that her sister's family was making such a courageous adjustment.

Andrew had always admired Louise, not only for the many kind things she had done for his family, but especially for her ability to lend her sister the strength to meet adversity. She had been a tower of strength for Mary Elvira, and on many occasions when they were still in Kansas she had also given Andrew encouragement when the public was particularly critical of his work and behavior. Her faith in his effort to improve the practice of medicine never wavered. It had been the support of the entire Hulett family that had sustained the Stills through some of their darkest hours.

It was early in the fall of 1880 before Andrew, now known affectionately by the public as the Old Doctor, was able to open his branch office in Hannibal. After he had investigated several sites in the city, was opened a small office on the north side of Broadway, between Ninth and Tenth Streets.

He had already treated patients from that part of the state, so it did not take long before he had a growing local practice. Patients from adjacent counties, as well as many of the local people, were clamoring for his help.

Some local doctors began to resent this unorthodox individual who was draining patients from their own practices. One Dr. Hearn was so disturbed by this maverick that he went to the Justice of the Peace and swore out a complaint, obtaining a warrant to prevent Andrew from practicing medicine in Hannibal without a license. George Mahan was the prosecuting attorney at that time and was not too interested in prosecuting this complaint. He felt it was more persecution than prosecution. He had several friends and neighbors who had been helped by Dr. Still's treatments and he felt this new type of treatment might benefit many people in his community.

Mahan tried to talk Dr. Hearn out of going to trial, but was unable to get him to drop his charges. On the day of the trial, Andrew suggested that neither of them use a lawyer, but act as their own lawyers. Upon the recommendation of the prosecutor, the judge agreed to this unusual procedure.

Andrew calmly described his background in practice and described the method he used to treat the sick. He explained how it offered help for conditions that would not respond to regular medical treatments. Dr. Hearn, on the other hand, launched into an angry attack upon Andrew, calling him a faker and charlatan. After this character assassination, the jury was so alienated that it quickly ruled in favor of Dr. Andrew Still. When asked later, Prosecuting Attorney Mahan was not exactly sure of the date of this trial, but thought it was in 1881.

Though there would be times in the future when some of his students would be brought into the courts, Andrew Still, as founder of this new science, was the first to be summoned before a court of law for practicing these new methods.

With all the publicity this trial brought to Hannibal, Andrew's office was soon too small to take care of the increased load of patients. With so many patients in Kirksville and so many from other towns requesting his services, Andrew finally decided to abandon his branch office.

Actually, the trial in Hannibal would have been unnecessary if Dr. Hearn, who initiated the case, had only waited a little longer. In his anger, he had failed to notice that Dr. Still was already making plans to close his branch office. Keeping the office in Hannibal and traveling back and forth from his home in Kirksville was not financially feasible nor an effective use of his time.

With his court experience before a jury, Andrew had learned more about how to present his new discovery to the public and to the medical community. He had always felt he was on the threshold of a great discovery and with a greater variety of patients to help him expand his knowledge he grew more confident in treating a wider range of conditions.

If his theory was correct, there must be some mechanical factor preventing the free flow of blood, lymph, and cerebral spinal fluid as a causative basis for body malfunction and disease. Finding this specific structural abnormality was essential to the treatment of any pathological condition that resulted from stasis.

For the past few years, he had had the opportunity to treat nearly every kind of disease that afflicted humans, except insanity. After closing his office in Hannibal and visiting briefly with his family, he was allowed to treat mental patients in the State Hospital at Nevada, Missouri. After seeing several types of mental illness and treating them, he became convinced many cases could be improved and some actually cured using his methods. However, the demands on his time were becoming so great that he was not able to spend as much time in Nevada as he would have liked in order to do follow-up work with the patients he had treated.

As busy as he was, he could have used help. But his own boys were still too young to be trained to treat patients and he also felt they should have a background in anatomy and physiology before they even considered following in his footsteps. So, as an experiment, he decided to take two other young men under his wing: one was a strong farm lad, the other a slightly better educated youth who had expressed an interest in learning from the Old Doctor. For about three months, they followed him around, trying to grasp what he was doing.

The farm boy quickly discovered that what looked so simple when applied by the skilled hands of Andrew Still was impossible for him to do or understand. The other young man stayed a bit longer, but soon he told Dr. Still it would be a lot easier for him to just go to medical school where he could learn from textbooks how to treat sick patients. So Andrew lost his first two students: one to the farm and the other to medical school. However, he had learned that the complexities of his approach to disease would require a comprehensive knowledge of anatomy and physiology before anyone wishing to do what he was doing could grasp the technique.

During a period of three or four years, Andrew had seen patients in nearly every town in northern Missouri and had been invited to Kansas City. He had even been invited back to Baldwin where he had had such unpleasant experiences, and to Arkansas where some of the towns that had been built around natural springs had become a mecca for the sick and infirm.

It soon became obvious that with the volume of patients he was seeing, it would be wise to just stay in his hometown of Kirksville and have his patients come to him there. He was thrilled that people would come to him in such large numbers for his services. He often had to reserve all the rooms in all the largest hotels in Kirksville to accommodate even a fraction of the patients clamoring to be seen by the now well-respected Dr. Still.

His wife and friends finally persuaded him not to try to do more than his strength would bear. Even with all this persuasion, in the beginning he only decided to curtail his travels and, even then, only after he had decided to build some form of infirmary in Kirksville.

In all his travels, one place he had avoided for several years was Macon, the town where he had first planned to make his home after moving from Kansas. He had often wondered why the Methodist preacher had been so adamantly opposed to him since he had helped quite a few patients in that community during his short stay there.

His brother Edward, who still lived in Macon, had finally become interested in Andrew's type of practice and visited him in Kirksville occasionally to exchange ideas as well as to get a better understanding of Andrew's concepts. One day Andrew finally brought up the subject of why the Macon preacher had made it so hard on him even though he had been doing a fairly good job with the sick.

Edward told his brother that the Methodist preacher who had caused him so much trouble had recently left Macon, but before leaving he told Edward that shortly before he made the vicious attack on Andrew, he had received a letter from the preacher in Baldwin who reported some of the ugly rumors that had been circulating in Douglas County – that Andrew was in league with the devil, that he was a midnight-walking grave-robber who would be capable of terrorizing people wherever he lived. Edward told Andrew that the preacher was so afraid of him because he was a satanic individual and that he felt he must do everything in his power to force him to move away.

Andrew was not too happy that his brother had not shared this information with him before, and he still was not too pleased that his brother hadn't been more helpful when he had returned to Missouri and so needed his help, but he decided that he might as well put this in the past and forget it. Besides, Edward was beginning to use some of the brains he had been born with and was showing signs that he was beginning to grasp some elements of Andrew's new concepts.

Even with his failure to impart his new concept to the two young men who followed him for a while, Andrew was convinced that his science and method could be taught. He had taken his sons Charley and Harry on trips with him and demonstrated the relationship of anatomical changes to physical infirmities. He had then shown his sons how it was possible to correct these conditions.

Though they were good observers, Andrew realized the boys would need basic education before they could grasp his concept and be of real assistance to him. He spent quite a bit of time thinking about how he could provide proper education for them so that his new science could be developed and expanded. Being growing boys, they were not always interested in, nor even aware of, their father's plans for the future.

Charley had always been involved in sports, especially baseball. When he accidentally learned to throw a curveball – none of his fellow players had ever seen such a pitch before – he spent nearly all his time away from school improving his discovery and developing control of his pitches. Soon he was throwing a big roundhouse curve and giving the local batters all kinds of trouble. It wasn't too long before town teams in the area were offering him money to pitch against their rival teams.

Herman was bitten by a travel bug, and once the family grew less dependent upon money from him, he took summer jobs in Illinois, spending increasingly more time away from home.

Harry, Herman's twin, in contrast was more of a homebody. He often said the reason he spent so much time with his father was that, left alone at home, he almost always got into trouble. All the children had heard many unkind remarks about their father the entire time they were growing up, and Harry became so emotionally upset when his father was referred to as a "crazy crank," that he was constantly involved in fights to defend Andrew's name. Harry was large and combative and he had a great deal of success in stopping the ugly remarks with his fists. Finally, Andrew decided to take Harry with him on as many trips as possible to keep him away from his tormentors.

The two younger children, Fred and Blanche, were also bothered by the things they heard about their father, but Blanche suffered most acutely during the periods of poverty the family had experienced. Not only was she forced to wear poorly made clothes, but for a time the other children teased her about wearing clothes made from flour sacks. Although her mother had many abilities, being a seamstress was not one of them. For Blanche, these periods of poverty in her formative years and hearing the unkind things said about her father were to stay with her throughout her life. While her brothers were able to forget, Blanche could not. Her memories colored her life with some bitterness.

Charley still accompanied his father on some trips, but much of his time was taken up with his new love, baseball. Gradually, Harry became the one his father turned to when he needed a helper and companion. Although Andrew had hopes that his children would all be able to be involved in his new system of treatment, he knew it was normal for them to have other interests. Nonetheless, there were times when he felt that the others could have been more available and useful in his work. His work load was increasing; there was a constant demand that he see more and more patients. He had reached a point where he knew he shouldn't travel so much, but requests from more and more places were hard for him to turn down. Even with his growing practice, he continued to treat many without charge and with his earnings from paying patients were often shared with those he considered worse off than himself.

For the next few years there were promoters and "money managers" who saw the financial potential of this new type of treatment, and they were eager to offer Dr. Still a considerable amount of money if he would allow them to take over the management of his services and put his entire operation on a sound financial footing. Some of these men were simply promoters who did not have the skill or background to be of much help. However, there were at least two men who were quite capable of creating a "money making" organization. One gentleman from Boston wanted Andrew to move to the East

Coast and offered him the guarantee that the Still family would have more money than it had ever thought of having before. This might have interested some members of the family, but it had no appeal to Andrew.

Andrew never had much use for money and strictly cherished his independence. He felt that many of his better ideas had been developed during his walks into the countryside or through the forest where he could commune with nature. As he thought about rejecting the offer to move east, he gave his sense of humor free rein.

He looked in the mirror and thought, "What would the Bostonians think of a doctor attired in a blue flannel shirt without a collar, a black slouch hat that had seen better days, and disreputable corduroy pants stuffed into worn boots?" This thought was highly amusing to him.

There were times when the idea of turning down so much money was not a happy one to others in the family. But they certainly were not surprised about his decision, knowing how he valued his independence more than anything that money could buy. By this time, the boys had learned that their father was a very special person. The family knew it was going to take quite a bit of help from all of them to allow him to fully develop his new science. Mary Elvira was such an unselfish helpmate that her dedication had rubbed off, in varying degrees, on all the children.

The boys thoroughly enjoyed teasing their mother. On one occasion, she bought a young bull when she thought she had bought a heifer. The boys kidded her about this error for years, but in later years, when Andrew was finally receiving so much praise, the boys were very vocal in expressing their opinion that if it hadn't been for their mother, there would not have been a discovery or the development of this new science.

By the mid-1880s Mary Elvira found it increasingly difficult to keep her husband from working too hard. Also, he was getting such attractive offers to see patients in so many places that he never seemed able to enlarge his office or start an infirmary in Kirksville as he had wished. On many occasions she pleaded with him to conserve his strength and energy, but there were so many requests for his services from out of town that he continued to spend time on the road.

It was no real surprise, though it did come as something of a shock, when early in April 1885, Andrew rather suddenly became completely exhausted. His rupture became active once again, this time to such a degree that he was only able to do a very limited amount of practice. He was once again quite discouraged. As a result, he again wrote to the Committee on Pensions, pointing out that they had on file a previous request providing the information about how he had served and how he was injured. In a letter of April 22, 1885, he wrote:

> I would like to have your rating as I know you will do me justice and not stint, whether I am placed on the list of pensioners or not. You will find in my evidence now on file that I was an early volunteer in 1861 at Fort Leavenworth, Kansas. I have written this believing that the department did not understand the conditions under which I fought. I was either a Missouri or a United States soldier when I left Kansas. If neither, I was an outlaw, for we killed nearly one-hundred men while in Missouri and thought we did so by the authority of the United States.

After waiting seven months and receiving no reply, on January 22, 1886, Mary Elvira wrote to the Committee on Pensions. The following are excerpts of her letter:

> Major General Curtis, as a U. S. officer, called for volunteers to go over into Missouri and help him and it was

during that fight over in Missouri under a U. S. officer that my husband was injured.

I think he is entitled to a pension. He has laid his case before many eminent lawyers. They all say it is a clear case and I hope in your generous rulings that you will say so too.

She then added:

I was appointed in December of 1861 as Matron of the hospital in Harrisonville, Missouri by Col. Nugent and served in that capacity until about April of 1862. I never realized a cent. Is there any way for me to get anything? Please tell me what steps I shall take and oblige.

On April 23, 1887, after a period of nearly twenty months, the assistant secretary to the Commissioner on Pensions wrote Andrew that his request was again denied and Mary Elvira didn't receive a reply to her letter at all.

In spite of the shabby treatment he had received, Andrew never wavered in his love of his country. He did at times question how it was being run by some of the politicians and department chiefs. He was particularly critical of the United States Army for the way it handled not only his request for a pension but those of his friends who had served with him in the Kansas Militia.

He felt quite a shock when two of his sons decided to enlist in the army in April of 1887. Charley and Herman signed up for a three-year tour of duty with the Fourteenth Infantry stationed at Fort Leavenworth, Kansas. Andrew was provoked that his sons had left him just as he was regaining much of his strength and his practice.

He and Mary Elvira were again in the middle of an effort to reorganize and felt they needed all the help they could get so that Andrew's mission could meet the demands now being placed upon him. His wife said that one thing was certain: she was going to be stricter in conserving Andrew's finite physical capacity this time.

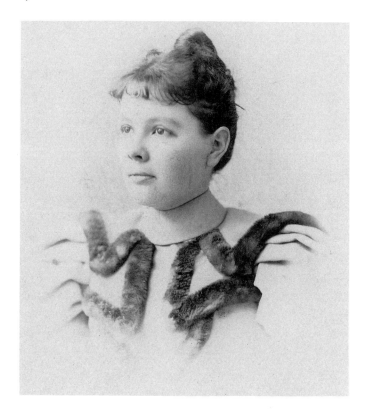

Anna Florence Rider (Mrs. Charles E.) Still

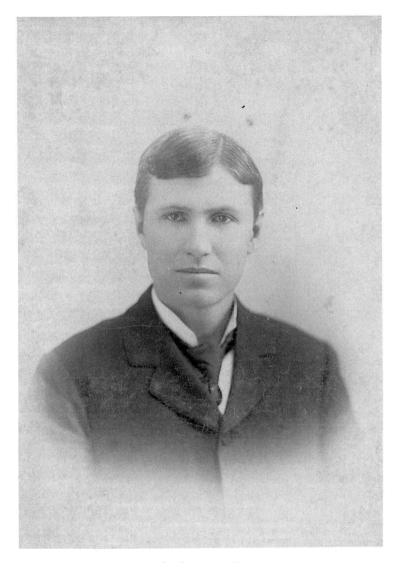

Charles E. Still

Chapter Nine

CHARLEY AND HERMAN felt bad about leaving their parents for such a long period of time and planned to send part of their army paychecks home each month so their mother would be able to pay the bills. It seemed to them that Harry was being groomed to be their father's number one helper, and they felt he was doing a first-class job. They also saw that Fred and Blanche were proving to be real helpers to their mother.

Before Charley joined the army, he had been seeing a young lady named Anna Rider. Her father, who had fought in many of the greatest Civil War battles, felt the Stills were too poor and didn't consider Charley a good match for his only daughter. When Anna and Charley began going together, Mr. Rider did everything he could to discourage them. When Charley left, Anna told him she would wait for him. She would change her father's mind, she assured him, by the time he finished his tour of duty.

The boys were assigned to different companies, so once they were in the service they didn't see much of each other. On payday, as planned, they sent their checks to their mother. While their pay was that of privates and so not much, it still meant they could contribute regularly to the family to help at home. During those years the regular army was not a place for rapid advancement. There were men in it who had held the rank of full colonel or higher in the Civil War who were now serving as lieutenants and captains.

WITH CHARLEY'S INTEREST IN BASEBALL, it didn't take long for him to become involved in army sports. At that time, there was quite a rivalry between the Infantry at Fort Leavenworth and the Cavalry at Fort Riley. For several years, the Cavalry had won in head-to-head competitions, much to the disgust of Brigadier General Alexander M. McCook.

When the general found out that Private Charley Still had pitched winning baseball for teams in Missouri, and had a new pitch that puzzled batters, he was thrilled, thinking he might now be able to break the domination of the Fort Riley Cavalry team. He had named his Infantry team "The McCooks" and had this name put on the uniforms.

The general was anxious to find out if the new pitcher was as good as he was rumored to be, so he scheduled a few games against the town teams in Kansas and western Missouri. Having no other method of transportation, the team was loaded into two horse-drawn ambulances and, since there was often no place to change clothes, the players traveled in their baseball uniforms. It was quite a sight to see more than a dozen young men, usually hot and sweaty, wearing baseball uniforms, pile out of the ambulances when they arrived at the field.

Charley had added a sharp-breaking curve to his assortment of pitches that made his roundhouse even more effective. This lengthened his winning streak. His Post could hardly wait for the next visit from the Fort Riley team. When the day finally arrived, Charley's curveball completely baffled the Cavalry batters. General McCook paced up and down the sideline during the entire game, shouting encouragement, or swearing when things went wrong. With the victory, the general forgot the dignity of his position and went out to the mound to give his young pitcher a hug and a slap on the back. With all of the attention he was getting, Charley began thinking of making the army his career.

While Herman was not enthralled with army life, he didn't mind some of the excitement that went with it. One instance that was quite a thrill for him was being at the land office when it opened in Guthrie, Oklahoma for the land rush. Sooners crossing into the territory before the specified time created a lot of excitement. He was happy to have a chance to be with his brother again and that they both were involved in this event (that would be chronicled in American history).

After the initial arrival of the Sooners, Herman's company spent time in Oklahoma trying to maintain order, while Charley's company was sent west along with other units to assist in trying to capture Apache Chief Geronimo who was mistakenly reported to be leading another Apache uprising.

As several units of the Fourteenth Infantry moved toward the West through the Oklahoma panhandle and into eastern New Mexico, many of the younger soldiers who had heard gory tales of Indian warfare lost the desire to catch up with this famous warrior. As the unit moved farther west, more and more frightened soldiers reported for sick call. Each day the number increased. The officers finally discovered that many of the stomach problems reported probably resulted from the fearful men's consumption of small quantities of soap.

While encamped in New Mexico and waiting for new orders, the troops tried to find ways to entertain themselves. Many men stayed with their poker games, but one of the new forms of entertainment was staging battles between tarantulas. There were often huge bets placed on favorites. Most of the men were not familiar with the large fuzzy spiders and had been told that the bite was always fatal, so the "fight to the death" of these huge spiders was not the only diversion. Some men discovered that when another soldier was concentrating on the spiders' death struggles he could be surprised if a large clod was dropped into one of his cupped hands. The victim of the joke would explode into action from his fear of the dreaded spiders. Sometimes he would react so intensely that, on a couple of occasions, some of the closer observers were actually pushed into the circle with the spiders. Because of the great fear of the tarantulas, a near riot would ensue whenever this occurred. The officers finally had to stop this form of entertainment before someone was crushed to death.

Charley's company of the Fourteenth Infantry spent nearly three weeks in New Mexico. The time passed slowly so the men were happy when they heard their services were no longer needed; the report of Geronimo's escape had been inaccurate. Now they could return to their home post. Although none of them saw any action against the Apaches, many later wore with pride the ribbon that indicated they were veterans of the Indian Wars.

A sore spot with Charley was that he hadn't heard a word from Anna Rider even though he had written her several letters. And while he was in New Mexico, he had written her about his adventures. When he arrived back at Fort Leavenworth, he expected to find a letter from Anna. But once again, the only letter awaiting him was one from his mother and sister that told of his Grandmother Still's death. He had always had great respect for his grandmother and admired the way she continued to live on alone in the old family home where he had been born. With only a little help from one of her daughters, she had been able to run the house and farm up until her death.

The second year in the army started off routinely for the Still boys with more than the usual amount of KP duty. One day while Charley was peeling potatoes, orders came to fall in: the name of a new corporal was to be announced. He was stunned when his name was called and he was asked to step forward. He thought he was going to be disciplined, but instead he was the private being promoted to corporal. He was truly surprised.

As pleased as he was with the promotion, he knew it was a mixed blessing. There were too many men who had served much longer than he who had been passed over. He was sure there would be some resentments, and this certainly proved to be true. On some occasions these veterans did things to make him look bad, but Charley did as good a job as possible and tried not to let their resentment bother him too much.

The baseball season was about to begin again and he knew past performances would not satisfy General McCook. This time the team would have to play the Cavalry at their home base, Fort Riley, and the Infantry would no longer have a friendly crowd. Instead, some of the toughest soldiers in the army would be trying to unnerve this young Infantry pitcher.

In preparation for this showdown, the Infantry played several teams from some of the larger cities. Pitching against a veteran team in Saint Joseph, Missouri, Charley's curveball had been particularly effective. Afterwards, a scout for a professional team from Kansas City talked to him seriously about becoming a professional ballplayer when he left the service. The confidence that he gained from his victories properly prepared him for the trip to face the Cavalry. There were other incentives for Charley as he fine-tuned his curve. The batboy on the team was the son of an army captain named Arthur MacArthur. The boy, named Douglas MacArthur, followed Charley around, amazed at the way Charley could bend his curveball. He often asked if, maybe, some day he could learn to throw such an unusual pitch. Another young "army brat," Orin Wolf, was the water boy. When the team left for Fort Riley, the players felt they couldn't let their army buddies down. They must also win for the two boys who so loved the team. (Young Douglas went on to become one of America's most famous soldiers and Orin Wolf became famous as one of the commanding officers in the Philippines during the capture of Aguinaldo.)

With such strong support, the Infantry team took the field with considerable confidence. The Cavalry was still unable to figure out how to hit Charley's curveball and when the McCook team left the field with their second straight victory over their vaunted foes, they were indeed a happy group. Perhaps the happiest were the batboy, MacArthur, and the water boy, Wolf.

Shortly after this game, Charley's picture appeared in the *Police Gazette* with an article about his pitching. This tabloid specialized in boxing, wrestling, and baseball. It wasn't the kind of publication seen in most homes but was found in barbershops and places where it had only a male audience.

Mary Elvira was aghast when someone brought a copy of the *Gazette* to her attention. She felt real embarrassment that her son's picture appeared in such a magazine. Andrew, on the other hand, half snorted and suggested it was about time for the boys to come home and help him with his growing medical practice. He had thought about buying the boys out of the service and bringing them home to help him, but since they were both adults he couldn't do this unless they agreed to it.

Andrew was dedicated to helping the sick and ailing in their battle to regain health, and knowing there were so many people needing his services made it hard for him to understand why his boys might not want to follow in his footsteps. His wife, however, knew the boys were individuals who might want to choose a life for themselves. Even though she was embarrassed by the article in the *Police Gazette,* she was proud that her boy had attained such success in baseball, which she knew he loved so much.

Charley and Herman had been home for three or four short furloughs. On each visit they had noticed the steady growth in their father's practice and realized that if they joined him they would have a great opportunity to be part of his expanding system for treating the sick and infirm. Andrew told his boys that in the near future he would find a way to see that they received proper training in his method of treatment and be provided, as well, with an education in both anatomy and physiology. The boys decided that since each had just one year left in their enlistment they might as well complete their remaining time in service. This would give their father time to set up the educational facility he had been discussing.

Herman had decided to join his father after his last furlough. Charley, on the other hand, had always wanted to be a soldier and had tried in vain to get an appointment to West Point before he joined the regular army. Recently he heard he might have an opportunity to go to Officer Candidate School. Liking army life, he had about decided that it would be the career for him.

It still bothered Charley that Anna had not written to him, nor had she been around on his brief visits home. It was true that her school was not in session on a couple of those occasions, but the one time she was in town she had made no effort to contact him. He had nearly concluded that she was purposely avoiding him.

Looking back, he remembered the first time they had met. It was at a revival meeting and they had joined the Methodist Church in Kirksville at the same time. Almost immediately, they started attending church together. He had told her that he had a job that paid very little. She had told him that wasn't very important to her. Over the dozen or so times they had attended church together and gone together to church picnics, he had assumed she was really interested in him.

When she came to the train to see him off to the army, she had told him that if he would write, she would love to correspond with him. Now, after two years and no word from her, he doubted her sincerity. Even so, he couldn't help but wonder why she had so carefully avoided seeing him.

Back at Fort Leavenworth, Charley was receiving lots of attention with the baseball season coming up. Now that many of the soldiers had won money from the Cavalry troop on their bets, baseball was becoming a hot item of interest. General McCook had invited several good semipro teams to play against his now well-publicized team. Not only had the pitcher had his picture in the *Police Gazette,* but the first baseman had also made that tabloid. He, too, had been offered a professional contract. (He later made it into the Big Leagues.)

Nearly all the games attracted large crowds, but a new wrinkle in baseball teams brought out an overflow crowd. A team of "Bloomer Girls" was touring the Midwest, and although the quality of their play left quite a bit to be desired, several of them were very attractive and had enough athletic skills to play a fair game against the average small town team. The Fort Leavenworth team now was a well-seasoned outfit with several outstanding players, especially a pitcher who could throw a curveball. The Bloomer Girls were definitely outmatched, but they still thrilled the crowd of young soldiers.

Corporal Still, who had been listening to baseball scouts offering him professional contracts, felt a bit embarrassed when he took the mound against these young women. He tried to throw a straight fastball without much "mustard" on it. He also mixed it in with a change-up that he had been working on lately. The crowd of soldiers in the stands kept calling for his famous curve ball. Not wanting the young women to look bad, or maybe get hit by his pitch, he decided to throw the curveball at half speed.

Although he had taken a bit of speed off his curveball in the past, this time he threw it with such a strange motion that he felt something snap in his shoulder. He was barely able to finish the game. He knew he had done something to his pitching arm that might be quite serious.

With the game against the Cavalry only a few weeks away, he was really worried about how he would be able to perform against such a good team with an arm that could not throw that sharp-breaking curve ball. It didn't hurt so bad when he threw his fastball, which was never exceptional, but he could not make his best pitch break in its usual fashion. He knew what was expected of him; he also knew that nearly everyone in camp would be betting his paycheck on the outcome of the game; and he was certain General McCook would not tolerate a loss to the Cavalry unit. Most of all he knew the batboy and water boy would be unhappy if he failed them.

For several weeks he kept trying to get his shoulder loosened up so he could throw his best pitch, but as hard as he tried, it was not to be. He had never worked too hard to develop a good change-up, but since his sharp-breaking curve was out of the question, he spent as much time as possible trying to master a good off-speed delivery.

The game was to be played in front of all his friends and supporters. When he had taken the mound before, he had been blessed with a feeling of confidence. This time, he felt completely empty as he faced the first batter.

For three innings, he was able to spot his fastball, and with some good fielding support the Cavalry hadn't gotten a man on base. In addition, his teammates had given him a couple of runs to work with. The next three innings were nearly disastrous for the Infantry team. Four long doubles in the fifth and sixth innings brought in two runs, and if it hadn't been for some fine defensive plays, the game would have been broken wide open.

Having lost a little speed from his fastball, and facing the last three innings in a tie game, Charley began using his change-up. Much to his surprise, the Cavalry team was still looking for that sharp-breaking curve and were way out in front of many of his pitches.

Luckily for the McCooks the team was still tied, 2-2, at the start of the ninth. Charley's arm and shoulder were stiffening and he doubted he could pitch another inning. He was also the second batter in the last of the ninth. When the first batter "popped up," things didn't look so good for the home team.

Charley, like many pitchers, was never considered a good hitter, nor had he ever gotten a hit off of Fort Riley pitchers. When he came to bat, he always got a round of jeers from the opponents because he batted cross-handed. This time the Cavalry "jockeys" were really giving him fits. They knew he was wearing down and if they could go into extra innings they were fairly sure of winning.

After a couple of feeble swings, the home crowd was deathly quiet as the visiting pitcher wound up. The batter was so jammed by the pitch, that it "squirted" down the third base line fair and Charley was able to stumble all the way to second base. A wild pitch and a long fly ball allowed the winning run to score.

Three victories in three tries established this young Corporal as quite a favorite. Not only General McCook, but nearly everyone on the Post was toasting the team pitcher. The young batboy and water boy had tears of joy running down their faces.

Charley took a bow after scoring the winning run, but he knew he would probably never be able to pitch again and that his chance as a professional baseball player was gone. He ruefully thought, "Well, this certainly has helped me decide to stay in the army. Hopefully, I can become a commissioned officer and have a secure future ahead." Knowing that Herman was going back to help his father reduced Charley's feeling of guilt about not being one of the cogs in building a new branch of medicine.

But he still wondered about his "girl" back home. He felt sure she cared for him. He thought that if he could see her again, since his interest in her wasn't being reciprocated, perhaps the feeling for her would go away. He requested a fourteen-day furlough and went back to Kirksville wearing a brand new army uniform. He made up his mind to find Anna, determine how she was, and ask her point-blank why she had not answered his letters.

The first thing he found out when he got home was that his father was actually going to start his school during the next year. And he learned his father had finally named his new science – he called it Osteopathy.

Charley told his father, "There's no such word in the dictionary."

Andrew replied, "Well, there's going to be!"

The county fair was in progress, so Charley spruced up and joined the crowd. Shortly he spotted that pretty country girl he had not seen nor heard from in nearly three years. When she saw him, she smiled, and soon they were walking together.

He asked her why she hadn't written him and learned she hadn't received a single letter he had sent. It took Charley very little time to figure out that her father had destroyed all those letters he'd written her. He felt he could never forgive Anna's father for trying to prevent them from seeing each other.

On their walk, she asked if he was coming back to help his father or returning to an army career. He admitted that he had about decided to become an officer and stay in the service. Seeing this fresh-looking young woman, though, made him less sure of his decision.

The next ten days of his furlough moved ever so slowly for Corporal Still. He had been so certain that he had correctly chosen a career in the army. He had also been sure that after he saw Anna again he would be able to remove her from his thoughts and dreams. But things were not developing the way he had planned. Anna's naturally curly hair, pleasant smile, and ability to talk with him seriously, as well as her interest in his father's work, made him think about what a good wife she would make.

Charley had also been having some long talks with his mother. He knew his father was soon starting a school in which his children and other interested young people would have an opportunity to study anatomy and physiology. With that foundation, they could then be taught more about his science of Osteopathy and they would understand it better.

People were convinced that the treatment the Old Doctor was using could not be taught, but Andrew's sons knew this was not true. They had all been able to help patients with a variety of conditions under their father's supervision, and they had even helped a few cases that their father had never seen.

Mary Elvira was quite frank when she spoke to her eldest son about his father's need for him. She pointed out that although Harry had been the one working with Andrew while Charley and Herman were in the army, every son would be needed once the school was opened. There were roles that each could handle: Harry was well qualified to handle the financial requirements; Herman probably had more mechanical skills and might be able to absorb his father's structural concepts more rapidly than the others, but his tendency to take off unexpectedly and be gone for a week at a time would probably not be too helpful; and Charley, she said, had the ability to get along well with people and he would be a real asset when they finally set up their institution.

Andrew was provoked that the two boys had gone into the army, so he said very little to them about the school. He knew Herman would return; he hoped Charley would. He felt worst about Charley because Charley had been such a help during the early days – he wasn't going to beg him to do anything.

Charley talked with quite a few people during this furlough, including a couple of lawyers who were dubious about Andrew's founding a medical school since they, like other people, were convinced that Osteopathy, as a science, was too individual to be taught to others.

Charley wondered what assurance he would have if he gave up his promising army career to learn his father's science and practice something that had no legal status. He was well aware of the many legal battles his father had endured. When his furlough ended and he headed back to Fort Leavenworth, he knew if he was going to pursue his goal of becoming an army officer he would have to reach that decision soon.

At least part of his time on this furlough had been pleasant and exciting. Every evening, he and Anna, whom he now considered "his girl," took long walks together. She listened intently to his army experiences and was thrilled to hear about his baseball successes and his chance to become an officer. She told him one reason her father was allowing her to spend so much time with him was that he knew Charley would soon leave permanently for the army.

It was difficult for Charley to believe that this young lady whom he hadn't seen for such a long time was so quickly becoming a big part of his life – and part of the entire Still family's life, too. She was so interested in how Charley's mother had held the family together during their lean times and she seemed to revel in the recent successes and accomplishments of the Old Doctor.

On the afternoon of the day before Charley was to return to Kansas for the final three months of his enlistment, he and Anna took a long walk together. They had talked about many things during the two-week period, but they had never said much about their budding romance or their future plans. They were about to finish their walk when Anna stopped and turned to her "man in uniform" and said, "Are you planning to come back to Kirksville to help your father or are you going to stay in the army?"

To his surprise, Charley heard himself say, "There is only one person in the world who could influence my decision."

She said, "Well, I would like to do anything I can to help you."

"You are the only person who can do it," he replied.

She looked slightly puzzled and repeated, "I will do anything I can."

Charley took her hand, looked into her eyes and said, "Name the day."

Charley's mother and the rest of the family were delighted to hear the good news – that he would be back home and out of the army in three months and that he would be marrying Anna.

It is doubtful that this came as good news to Captain Louis Rider, but at least he would have his daughter at home for an additional eight months, for the date Anna had chosen for her wedding was the thirtieth of June of the following year.

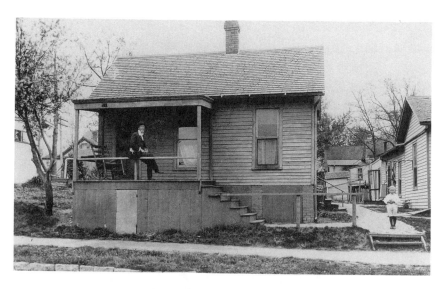

First School of Osteopathy

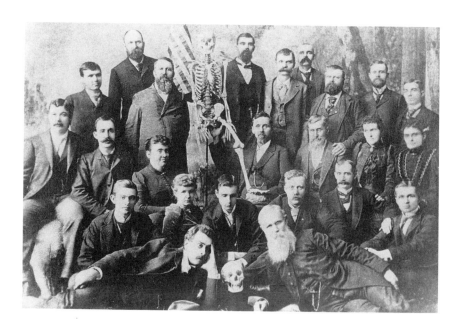

First Graduating Class of Osteopathy

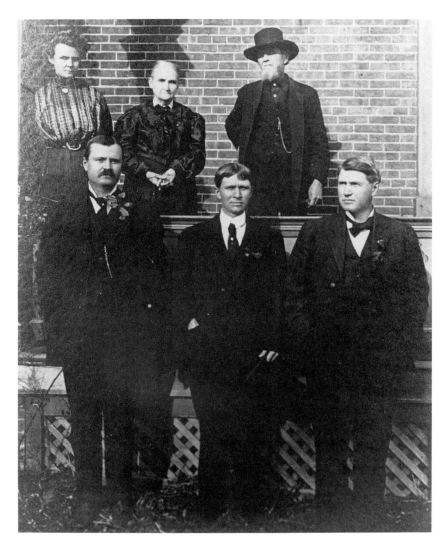

A. T. Still Family

Chapter Ten

Y THE FIRST OF JANUARY, 1892, the entire Still family was back together and anxious to see that Andrew got his school started, but with so many patients to see and so much time spent on the road, it appeared that he wasn't making much progress. While Andrew was visiting Eldorado Springs, where he had built up a large practice, three medical doctors there reminded the Old Doctor that he had promised them he'd have his school in operation that year. The doctors – Ward, an eclectic physician; Hatton, an allopath; and Davis, a homeopath – were anxious to enroll in his institution as soon as possible.

AS SOON AS CHARLEY RETURNED to Kirksville from the army, his father told him to hurry and get a charter for the school. Charley was puzzled. He didn't know what to ask for, nor did he have any idea what procedure to follow to obtain such a charter. Nonetheless, he approached Judge Ellison and asked for help in securing the charter.

The judge looked Charley directly in the eye and said, "Young man, your father is a gifted man, but when he dies, his system will die with him."

Charley told the judge that he himself had successfully treated patients that his father had never seen. The judge remained unconvinced.

He said, "Charley, where would your father teach?"

"Judge, I really don't know," he replied.

The judge asked one more question. "Who would do the teaching?"

Charley again had to tell the judge he did not know.

"What kind of curriculum would the school have?" the judge asked.

Charley had to tell the judge that they weren't too sure of that either.

After working with a young lawyer for a few weeks, they were able to develop a document that, with a few changes by the judge, would serve as the charter they so badly needed.

With the charter in hand, but with no faculty or buildings, it would take a real stroke of luck to make things move ahead. About this time, a young graduate in medicine from the University of Edinburgh arrived in Kirksville. He was working for a surgical supply company from Saint Louis. He spent some time and had some drinks with some of the local M.D.'s who told him about this old "crank" who had about ruined their practices and continued to fool many people.

This was certainly a challenge for the young Dr. William Smith. He was certain that after he quizzed Dr. Still with the right questions, he could show him up as a faker. When the two first met, Dr. Smith threw a long series of his best questions at Andrew regarding anatomy, physiology, and the best methods of diagnosing many different conditions. He discovered that this frontier doctor had most of the right answers and although he had come to ridicule, he found himself being converted, instead, to Andrew's beliefs. Now he only hoped that perhaps he could soon become a student of this doctor who, through his powers of observation, had learned to use the inherent laws of nature to create a new system of medical thinking.

As he reviewed his interview, Dr. Smith realized he had talked to a man who had learned much about the ability of the body to maintain its own health if it were given assistance in freeing up its untapped capabilities. The human body had all of the chemicals and disease-fighting material, even drugs, to control pain, and an immune system designed to repel infection.

Following their long discussion, Dr. Smith spent a restless night in his hotel room. He had decided to make a major change in his life. Instead of traveling from one large town to the next, visiting and even socializing with local doctors, he would now be living in a town without paved streets, and would be teaching anatomy, perhaps to a very heterogeneous group of students. In addition, he had no assurance of financial reward.

Dr. Smith continued to marvel at how the Old Doctor had been able to gain such a grasp of anatomy without the benefit of first-class formal instruction. He was also deeply impressed that Dr. Still claimed that he was only beginning to understand the scope of his new discovery. Andrew compared Osteopathy to "a squirrel in a tree with his tail sticking out and most of his body still in the tree, waiting to be pulled out." Dr. Smith was happy that he would be able to assist the founder of Osteopathy in his quest.

The Still home had become a beehive of activity: Herman helped his father supervise the building of the small frame structure that proved to be too small even before it was completed. Harry helped his father plan how the school's financial needs would be met and, if the school were enlarged later, how that need could be anticipated.

The addition of Dr. Smith to the faculty to teach anatomy left Andrew free to teach not only the practice of Osteopathy, but his own approach to physiology as well. Charley was assigned to interview prospective students and to look for qualified instructors. Finding additional faculty at that time was an impossible assignment. Who in his right mind would jeopardize a career in order to join a new and unproven profession and a school that might not make it through its first year? It was rumored that if the school actually got started, the medical profession was already organizing a move to place a bill in the Missouri Legislature that would prohibit the teaching of this drugless system, or cult, as they called it.

One thing that did please the Old Doctor was that women as well as men were enrolled in his first class. He had watched his well-educated wife struggle when they needed money and the most she could do was sell magazines and get odd jobs. Even teaching paid women very little. It had always been one of his goals to establish Osteopathy as a career open to women, too. He could envision that Osteopathy would offer a good livelihood and he made a point to see that women had every opportunity to have the same access to this career as the men. As a further incentive to women, he had lowered their tuition to about half that of the men. Also, being a strong abolitionist, he hoped that individuals of all races would have access to his school.

On October 3, 1892, at 10:00 A.M. Dr. Still and Dr. Smith began teaching seventeen students crowded into a building that lacked most of the comforts of modern life. These students had come to learn. And they had two great teachers.

Dr. Smith, with nothing more than a skeleton and a copy of *Gray's Anatomy,* made his subject so vibrant that many students felt they could visualize the total body and its functions as well. The Old Doctor was able to impart his confidence in the ability of the body to meet the stresses of living if it were given an opportunity to function, unhampered by structural interferences or injury.

This first student body ranged in age from eighteen to sixty-five. These students immediately felt they had started on an exciting, uncharted voyage with the Old Doctor guiding them to a new and promising opportunity and with Dr. William Smith as first mate.

The enthusiasm that Andrew felt – and instilled in his students – made the work load of teaching and seeing so many patients less of a chore. There were some students, however, who were unable to grasp the basic concepts of Osteopathy and this sometimes discouraged him and made him feel that he should not have started the school in the first place.

There was something else that really worried the Old Doctor: If his school were to grow and prosper, his son with the most financial sense should be in charge. During the time that Herman and Charley had been in the army, he had groomed Harry for that assignment. But there was one problem with putting Harry in charge. He had been less able than the other boys to cope with the criticism heaped on his father during his growing years. As a result, even though he was always able to manage money, he lacked the confidence to be a good administrator.

Early in 1892, even before the school started, Andrew had written a note to Harry: "You are a natural financier. Get a hold on the purse strings, as your brothers can break The Bank of England without any help. I must get out of practice and worry soon. Take charge of the business. If you cannot control the finances, step down and out, or else you will lose what little you have accumulated."

Neither Herman nor Charley had shown ability to handle money and both at times spent money like it was going out of style. But they had developed a bit of mental toughness and an ability to get along with people, characteristics that were so necessary in dealing with a variety of individuals. Charley also had been thrust into a leadership role when he served as captain of his baseball team. Herman never liked to accept responsibility on a day-to-day schedule, but could be a real help on a part-time basis.

When the organization of the school was completed, Andrew was the president, Charley was vice president, and

Harry was secretary and treasurer with complete control of the finances. The school was set up as a stock company with the immediate Still family holding the controlling shares, and other family members sitting on the board of directors. This freed Andrew from administrative duties so that he could do what he loved to do – teach. He would also have time to see patients, now arriving in Kirksville on a daily basis, who were suffering from some of the most difficult conditions and illnesses.

Andrew had often spoken of cutting down his practice and his teaching load, but instead he was working even longer hours with the stimulation of such a variety of conditions to challenge his skills. He always combined his treatment with instructional lectures to patients, feeling that if they had a better understanding of their problems, as well as what he was trying to accomplish, it would help them make a better recovery.

As he presented cases before his first class of students he discussed the abnormality that existed and he went into some detail regarding the anatomy and physiology that was involved in each case. He would sometimes have a student or two hold the patient in the proper position while he would explain exactly what he was doing and why. He had developed a real skill in choosing the right words and terms so that the patient would have a good idea of what was being done. Andrew's skillful teaching, in turn, made it simple for his students. He could explain and sell Osteopathy to his patients in such a clear way that many who were exposed to his teaching methods were later able to go out into the world and convince the uninformed about the value of this new science.

Despite his ability to create a nearly religious enthusiasm in his students for their profession and its potential, there were some students who worried the Old Doctor. He realized they would never have the understanding or the ability to practice as competently as Osteopaths. Although he was a tolerant and understanding man, he had great difficulty when someone asked him the same question over and over again. It was this type of student who as a graduate might do harm and bring a bad name to Osteopathy. He could not think of a way to keep this new profession free from incompetents. There was no way to screen an individual carefully enough to guarantee the finished product. Although he thought seriously of closing his school, there was such momentum going that, despite misgivings, he agreed to continue for at least another year. There was also such an increase of patients and potential students that it would have been most difficult to stop, or even slow down, the expansion.

As pleased as Andrew was about the growth of his profession, the demand for more space for new students, and the expansion of facilities to house new patients who were coming to Kirksville and staying for several months of treatment, he realized that there must be a lot of decisions made and soon. Probably the most important one had to do with the best use of his family. Harry certainly had the financial brains of the family, but he found it a real chore to deal with the everyday problems that arose in running the institution. He was always such a worrier that at times it had an adverse effect on his co-workers. Charley, on the other hand, was able to handle minor issues without getting upset. But again, he had not shown a capability for handling financial matters. Herman disliked being tied down by routine and would often disappear for a few days without giving notice to anyone. Fred was young and inexperienced, and his health had failed following an accident. Blanche was helping her mother and also attending classes.

Along with the decision to continue the school and expand it as well came an immediate need for new faculty and staff members. There were other questions, too: How much faculty would be needed as more students enrolled? How many more would be needed in a couple of years if this growth continued? Andrew wished he had someone to help him make these decisions. He and Mary Elvira had long talks about these new situations that had to be dealt with on nearly a daily basis. Sometimes, the pressure of growth nearly overwhelmed them.

It had been such a short time since the local people had considered them as merely some sort of strange characters. Now, they not only accepted the Stills, but were often more than willing to assist them. These same local people often told Andrew and Mary Elvira that they had always had faith in their chances of success and that they wanted to be a part of it. Sometimes Andrew was amused by this outpouring of offers of help from these people he considered to be brand-new supporters. His wife and some of the children found it hard to stomach this sudden interest in the Still family and doubted the sincerity of this band of well-wishers who had so recently surfaced.

It was certainly true that the town of Kirksville had profited from Andrew's success. There had been fewer than five thousand people living there when the school started. By 1894, two years later, with an infirmary to be built and a new hotel in the plans, as well as a new building to take care of the growing number of students, it was a "boomtown," that now found itself on the map of the United States. People from ever greater distances were now looking on the map to locate Kirksville, Missouri, the Home of Osteopathy. This growth came so fast that it was hard to plan for even the next year, let alone three or four years in the future.

Andrew had never been totally convinced of the idea to start a college. He may have done so mainly to see that his five children would be able to continue his work. He was now faced with the realities of figuring out what was needed to improve his school and bring it up to a high-quality institution without losing the basic principles of his science.

He had realized for some time that one year of instruction was certainly not enough. There must be more subjects in the curriculum. A real problem was now not so much finding quality faculty, for many now began to realize that the college was going to be successful. The problem was in finding teachers who could understand and accept the principles of Osteopathy well enough that there would be no detractors among his expanding faculty.

Andrew knew that if his profession was to attain respectability the school must have faculty members who were well-rounded and had a good reputation before they came to Kirksville. He also knew that since some of these new instructors would be coming from well-established medical schools, they would need to be indoctrinated in the principles of his science and would have to be broad enough in their understanding of Osteopathy that their teaching would incorporate both the best of their subject and the philosophy and substance of the material he was presenting in his daily lectures. If they only gave lip service to his concepts there would be big trouble down the road.

He also knew that another problem might be the students who had little background education but were well-steeped in Osteopathy and who were planning to stay and help with the school. He was afraid they might be looked down upon by more highly educated faculty members.

As the school was getting ready for its second year of operation, no one was prepared for the explosive expansion that now faced the Stills. There had been so little time for controlled growth that Andrew hadn't been able to plan properly on how he could add facilities and personnel and at the same time see that when space was added it would at least meet the needs of the next three or four years.

The personnel issue was the most critical. He knew that there were some people who were more interested in a "quick buck" than in learning the principles of his science. They wanted to learn just enough so they could then go out and say that they were qualified to practice Osteopathy. This presented a dilemma because there were no standards and no state laws to set up criteria. There was certainly plenty of potential for abuse of his system of therapy by both faculty and students since most of the new members of the faculty were also taking classes so they would qualify to earn a diploma.

There were many "diploma mills" selling certificates to untrained individuals in the field of medicine that Andrew hoped that only truly dedicated and qualified graduates of his school would represent his profession. He knew that with the moneymaking potential of his system it would be hard to control and especially difficult to protect the future of his discovery.

By adding faculty members slowly and spending as much time as possible seeing that they really understood all of his basic principles he hoped to instill loyalty in his graduates. He hoped that those who were best trained and those most interested in seeing that patients received excellent treatment would make it harder for imitators to compete.

Osteopathy was both an art and a science which required skills that couldn't be obtained from a textbook. Andrew hoped for graduates who had both the understanding of what they had been taught and a zeal to help humanity. They could then help to keep their own profession free from untrained imitators.

Although he was named vice president, Charley was functioning as acting president of the school. Interviewing prospective faculty and spending time looking over the plans for the new infirmary were occupying much of his available time. He really needed someone to help him manage the growth of the institution. Fortunately, Henry Patterson became available. He was appointed secretary-treasurer and business manager of the school. This in turn freed Harry so he could assist in some of the administrative duties as well as serve as financial advisor.

With every available room in town filled with patients waiting to see him for treatment, it was necessary for Andrew to have his three oldest sons treat patients after they had been examined by him. It soon became necessary for some members of the first class to see the many new patients who were arriving by the trainload.

Arthur Hildreth, a young man whose parents had been patients of the Old Doctor, and who had been raised close to town, also proved to be a most welcome addition to the young men who were now available to help treat the hundreds of patients.

Meanwhile, the Missouri Medical Association had not forgotten to see what they could do to stop the growth of this mushrooming competitor. During the spring of 1893, they had introduced a bill into the Legislature requiring that to practice Osteopathy a person must first attend and graduate from a medical college. With quite a bit of assistance from Andrew's satisfied patients, this bill was defeated.

Soon, the first article appeared in a metropolitan newspaper in Saint Louis telling about the development of this new system of treatment and reporting on the great number of people streaming into Kirksville. The reporter also wrote that there must be some value in what Dr. Still was doing, even though he wasn't sure what it was. He stated that he also couldn't understand why the Old Doctor was so opposed to the use of drugs.

Once it appeared that the school was organized and functioning smoothly, Andrew was interested in having one of his sons pioneer the practice of Osteopathy outside Kirksville. As a result, shortly after his marriage to Anna Rider and with the approval of his father, Charley became the first Osteopath, aside from the Old Doctor himself, to go into practice. He opened an office in Minneapolis, Minnesota, which almost immediately involved him in litigation. The local medical group had papers served to prevent him from practicing in their state without a medical degree.

Fortunately, Charley had gone to Minneapolis at the request of one of the most important businessmen in Minnesota, who had received considerable benefit from Charley's treatments in Kirksville. This man, Mr. Wernicke, the head of a large harvesting company, was the first patient that Charley treated strictly on his own.* Mr. Wernicke was so happy with Charley's treatment in Kirksville that he sent his foreman to the young doctor, who also benefited from his treatment. This double success had led Mr. Wernicke to invite Charley to Minneapolis to treat some of his personal friends.

Following their wedding at the end of June, Charley and Anna hurriedly prepared to leave for Minneapolis on the fifth of July. They had hardly completed their honeymoon when they checked into the Windsor Hotel and were told that Mr. Wernicke had already lined up more than a dozen patients and that he wanted some of them to be seen right away.

After seeing patients for only four days, Charley received a letter from the secretary of the Minnesota Board of Health in which he was advised to stop his unlawful practice or face prosecution. When the medical group filed the suit against Charley, Mr. Wernicke hired the best law firm in Minnesota to defend him. The attorney, F. F. Davis, told Charley he would handle any future letters from the State Board of Health.

July in Minneapolis was a most profitable one for the young couple. However, they were tiring of hotel living and when some men from Diamond Bluff, Wisconsin said they would guarantee at least twenty-five patients to start with if

---

*At about this time, many of the students were beginning to treat patients on their own in anticipation of leaving to start their own practices. The Old Doctor prevailed upon them to stay awhile longer to fine-tune their skills. Charley's success with Mr. Wernicke showed the others that they all had the potential for success in practice.

the couple would come there for at least a month, Charley and Anna obliged. They were glad to return to a small town, and their time in Diamond Bluff was both pleasant and profitable. Soon a contingent from Red Wing, Minnesota talked them into spending a month in their community. It was now the middle of October, and business was booming. Patients were coming from several of the surrounding communities.

During the second week in Red Wing, a prominent city leader by the name of Curtis came to see the young Dr. Still with a badly injured hip joint. After looking it over, Charley told Mr. Curtis that this was a most difficult case. If his father was free, he would like to have Mr. Curtis' injury seen by Andrew. Charley contacted the Old Doctor and was delighted that a trip to Red Wing could be arranged.

After the appointment had been made, several other important businessmen came along. Although it was a most difficult dislocation to reduce, the Old Doctor did so easily. Osteopathy suddenly gained a great many supporters in Minnesota.

Before Andrew headed home, he was asked if manipulation would help diphtheria, since there was an epidemic in the Red Wing area. He answered that he had treated many such cases successfully, and in the next few days Dr. Charley was called upon to treat several diphtheria cases. Fortunately, an assistant, Dr. Charles Hartupee, had arrived from Kirksville to run the office while Dr. Charley spent the next three weeks, day and night, with young diphtheria patients.

The secretary of the State Board of Health lived in Red Wing and filed a complaint that the young Osteopath had failed to report one of the new cases properly or on time. Although three different attempts were made to prosecute Charley while he was in Red Wing, they all failed when the prosecuting attorney refused to proceed.

The secretary of the State Board of Health was so incensed that he contacted the state Attorney General, requesting action. But since both the governor and the secretary of state had been treated by Charley, the attorney general would not follow up on the request.

With all of this support and publicity, Charley's practice grew by leaps and bounds. He had one assistant who was busy all the time, so Charley asked his father to send Harry up to help him, too. By now, the practice handled any kind of acute condition, as well as obstetric cases.

Harry, who had become an outstanding manipulator, had worked primarily on chronic conditions. Now, he was thrust into the chaos of an acute care practice and was finding it hard to adjust to all of this confusion. He did not know that Hartupee and his brother had been treating a few epileptic patients with some apparent success. One morning, he arrived at the office at the moment that two patients had seizures simultaneously in an office crammed to capacity with other acute care patients.

Harry had seen enough. He wrote a brief note that he was headed home. He returned home briefly, then went to Minneapolis, where he practiced for several months.

With such a large practice, Charley considered making Red Wing his home. A Minnesota newspaper had even written that "by the time Charley Still retires, he might be one of the wealthiest men in the state."

However, the Old Doctor had discovered during Charley's absence that Charley was the one with the administrative ability and he needed him back. The school and infirmary were entering a very critical period and no one else had the ability to handle the administrative duties. Andrew wrote that, although giving up such a lucrative practice would be a hardship, Charley was really needed back in Kirksville.

Charley and Anna hated to leave Red Wing and give up a practice that had brought them friends and money enough to afford luxuries, but their loyalty to Andrew and Mary Elvira, and the Osteopathic profession, led them to bid a tearful farewell to their friends and patients in Minnesota where they had spent their first year of marriage. They knew their new challenge would be to guide the school during its greatest period of expansion. Andrew had watched many from his first class become successful in the profession he had started and loved. Harry, who practiced briefly in Minneapolis, had also returned to Kirksville and was developing a very successful practice. Herman, whom the Old Doctor had considered to have the most mechanical ability of any of his children, as well as an intuitive quality that was very helpful in diagnosis, had meanwhile set out on his own to start a practice in Illinois.

Andrew had seen the first "brood of chicks" carry his therapeutic gospel quite a distance from Kansas where it started and northern Missouri where it matured. Before long, it would encompass the globe.

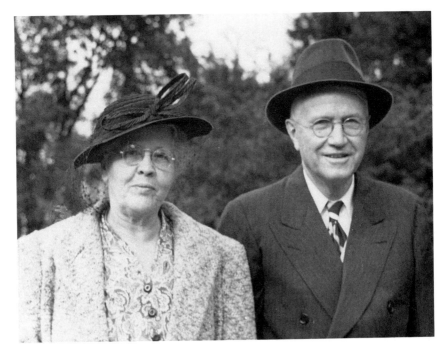

Dr. and Mrs. Charles E. Still

Chapter Eleven

S THE AMERICAN School of Osteopathy prepared for the fall of 1894, Andrew was gratified that Charley was back home to help with the many emerging problems. A year earlier Andrew had decided not to keep the school in operation, but he changed his mind and knew then that as soon as possible he must acquire a faculty that would give his students the basic education necessary to compete with graduates of other medical schools. He knew it would take some time to afford a highly qualified group of teachers, but he made the commitment to himself that it must be done. And soon.

He had been taking a hard look at the medical practices of the 1890s and the state of medical education. In the Midwest there were a number of medical "diploma mills" in operation. There was a disproportionate number of what he considered "second-class" medical schools, many of them in existence for less than five years. There was also a number of itinerant doctors who had never attended college and were now traveling from town to town, making exaggerated claims, and then moving on.

Since allopathic medicine was still the dominant therapeutic system, Andrew knew he must train his students well for the competition they would face when setting up practice. This goal would require special physical facilities such as a large building with enough space for classes, clinical services, and, hopefully, a laboratory and dissection program. If the program were to progress quickly, he must see that there was adequate housing for students and faculty. He was anxious to get the organization set up as soon as possible so he could achieve these goals quickly.

Harry arrived home to help plan the expansion of the school. He took over the construction of a hotel near the Wabash Railroad Station. Now patients who came from larger cities would find additional hotel space in Kirksville where they could stay long enough to receive full benefit of their treatments.

During that August, Andrew's nephew Thomas Still, his brother Edward's son who was an architect from Macon, designed the school's new infirmary building and began its construction. Andrew was surprised when his brother said he was thinking of entering the school when Andrew got it completely organized. Andrew had not forgotten the lukewarm support Edward had given him much earlier during his brief stay in Macon.

But Edward had since then spent quite a bit of time in Kirksville and sat in on some of the planning sessions for the new infirmary building. Andrew was prepared when he was called aside and Edward told him he had decided to enroll in the American School of Osteopathy in the near future. However, it was a real shock to Andrew when he received a letter from his brother Jim in Eudora. Jim wrote saying that he, too, was interested in attending the school. Andrew was glad his brothers had finally seen the light and could understand the value of his principles. He knew how hard it must have been for Jim to ask for this favor, especially after the way he had treated Andrew when he was in Kansas. It was difficult for Andrew to forget the letter Jim had written Edward at that time suggesting that it was dangerous to have a "crazy brother" as an associate. But now Jim, as well as Edward, had come around.

Although some of the present students were mature adults, they all considered the Old Doctor a father figure and called him "Daddy Still." It amused Andrew to think of his older brothers referring to him as "Daddy Still."

One of the women in the first class, Jeannette ("Nettie") Bolles, had done so well and set such a fine example that she was asked to join the faculty. Once it was proven that women could be good students, several others were ready to enroll in the next class.

In the meantime, Kirksville had begun to benefit from the school. For a town that hadn't grown much over the past decade, the sudden influx of visitors and the building boom the school inspired made the town fathers realize that the Osteopathy profession and its school were great assets.

There had been rumors going around town for some time that other towns, such as Des Moines, Kansas City, and Sedalia, were offering land, buildings, and money to Dr. Still if he would relocate his practice and school to their community. Hearing this, the Kirksville mayor and city council decided to see that Dr. Still stayed right there in Kirksville. Money was raised and land offered to keep the school.

Andrew felt a great sense of loyalty to Kirksville. His family was happy there and the community truly had accepted him. At the time that other city groups approached him, however, he was in no condition to review their offers. He was devastated by the death of his youngest son, Fred. His wife and daughter Blanche had taken Fred out west, hoping a change in climate would help his lung condition – an injury from a serious accident Fred had experienced earlier which caused his health to fail. A horse had pinned Fred against a wall of the barn, resulting in a splintered rib that punctured one of his lungs.

In spite of his deteriorating health, Fred had continued his studies and finished his class work before Andrew decided he would benefit from the move west. Andrew, as well as Fred's classmates, had always considered him a fine young man with an excellent mind. His death brought back vivid memories of the deaths of his other children years before in Kansas.

With the turmoil created by all the construction and by Fred's death, the Old Doctor spent even more time seeing patients and involving himself in the operation of the school. In addition, he devoted attention to formulating plans for the future of the college.

BY THE FALL OF 1894, there was a backlog of students waiting to enroll. Henry Patterson, secretary and business manager, said the school was not in any condition to take on additional students. He felt there were several hundred patients to be treated, which would require all available space and all of the staff's time. Not wanting to abandon the teaching program, however, Patterson finally agreed to allow a half-dozen students to start classes and a month later allowed nearly a dozen more to enroll. Understandably, confusion reigned during this time of expansion and growth.

Nearly all prospective students came from families who had directly benefited from Osteopathic services and who were eager to begin their schooling. There was also a great interest in learning as much as possible directly from the Old Doctor himself.

The students were an enthusiastic group. During their stay at the clinic they were exposed to the successes of treating such a variety of conditions that they were even more fervent about their future work. However, as eager as they were, some had doubts about their ability to practice on their own.

Even though the students saw the results of the treatment, much of it was under the supervision of the Old Doctor and many were worried that they might not grasp the theory of Osteopathy adequately to develop the skills that would make them successful in its practice.

The classes were often disorganized at this time and it is quite possible that some students might have given up and gone home had it not been for the friendliness of the Old Doctor and his family.

Through their work and their successes, Dr. Charley Still and Dr. Harry Still had demonstrated that the ability to achieve clinical results was not unique to Andrew, the Old Doctor, but that it could be taught to others. It was comforting for the students to know this. They knew the three Still boys – Charley, Harry, and Herman – had been tested under fire and had had successful practices. That they were there to help Andrew in training and teaching and in working with the patients further encouraged the students.

Living and breathing Osteopathy was essential for creating the enthusiasm and "fighting spirit" it would take to go out into the world and face opposition that was often formidable. There would be no laws or courts to protect them. It took the entire Still family to help students prepare mentally to carry the banner of Osteopathy to the four corners of the land and to face the doubters and organized opposition. These new Osteopaths were the ones to experience the trials which would later be called the "birth pangs" of the profession. It would require their dedicated pioneering spirit, while graduates of later classes would contend with the "growing pains."

Students in the first classes had the opportunity to meet and admire Mother Still, Mary Elvira, who had stood at the side of her embattled husband throughout some of the worst opposition any medical pioneer had ever faced. This exposure to those who had already been tested was a real help to the early students.

Andrew had passed his sixty-fifth birthday and, braced by the stimulation of his expanding profession, was ready to meet the new challenges of what proved to be the most productive decade of his life. He no longer had to use a cane or staff on his morning walks and the truss he had designed controlled his hernia. He continued to have the chest pain he blamed on the war and occasionally it was so severe he would have one of his students correct the rib problem that was producing the discomfort.

Since he often chose one of the new students to help him, he was asked at times why he had not chosen someone with more experience. He explained that the students who were least informed would follow his instructions better. He did, however, occasionally call in one of his sons to help him.

He liked to use his morning walks to prepare his lectures. He felt that the stimulation of being with nature helped him think more clearly. Since he started his classes at 6:30 in the morning, much of his walking was done while the stars were still out.

His lectures would last at least two hours. He always stressed the understanding of the total human body and the complete meaning of his Osteopathic philosophy. He felt that if one understood the normal structure and function of the body when faced with an abnormal condition, it should be possible to develop the best method to correct the abnormality and by the most appropriate means.

He was totally opposed to any treatment or correction that had any element of routine technique. He felt it would prevent the practitioner's thinking through each case on an individual basis, and he occasionally demonstrated this to students when presented with a particularly difficult case.

Sometimes, after a preliminary examination, he would sit motionless for as long as half an hour before trying to make any type of correction. Often the patient would become quite restless. Then Andrew would do what he thought was necessary. He explained this to his students, saying that he had to properly visualize the total condition before he could start to make a correction. One son related an incident in which the Old Doctor, on a house call, spent over an hour after his preliminary examination just sitting there with his eyes closed. The patient's family thought he was taking a nap and was displeased. When the Old Doctor finally made a very difficult correction, he left without offering any explanation. Andrew enjoyed the challenging cases and often assigned the routine cases to an assistant.

When 1894 began to wind down, it had proved to be one of the most important years for Osteopathy. The first class had graduated in March after completing a year-and-one-half course of study. Eleven graduating students received their diplomas at a ceremony in the Smith Opera House with President Dobson, of the local Normal School, serving as master of ceremonies. The program concluded with the presentation of diplomas and Dr. Still's address.

During the summer, the west part of Kirksville had expanded. Harry Still had started construction of the hotel near the railroad station with a groundbreaking ceremony on August 6, Andrew's sixty-sixth birthday. Construction had also been started on the new infirmary with Andrew's nephew Thomas in charge of design and construction.

Andrew prepared his graduates to be scrupulously honest in their dealings with the public. The first thing they must do, he said, was to avoid extravagant claims and they should stay in one area long enough to become known to the community. This was important, he stressed, because of the itinerant doctors who traveled from town to town making exaggerated claims for cures. Since Osteopathy was so new, he wanted his graduates to bring honesty, honor, and prestige to the profession.

Many early graduates entered practice in pairs because they needed the confidence of someone with whom they could share their problems and also to help them care for the many patients wanting to benefit from this new type of therapy.

Andrew always made himself available to the graduates who were starting their own practices. When his son Charley had had a difficult case, he had gone to Red Wing, Minnesota to help. Now, with most of his graduates within a hundred miles of Kirksville, he would often drop in to offer encouragement. With his reputation, the fact that he would take time to stop by a former student's office often gave the student's practice a boost, ensuring more rapid success.

Toward the end of 1894, the infirmary building was nearing completion and students and interested townspeople were invited to add bricks to its walls. Andrew enjoyed sharing his success with his friends and students, and this was one way in which they could all take an active part.

He considered his early students a part of his family and often spent special time with them. Some discussions they had were on how to handle problems other than physical ones which patients might have. He pointed out that not all patients could be cured, but that this in no way should prevent a doctor from giving them his best effort. He stressed that keeping the interest of the patient first was the key to managing a case. And sometimes, he said, the results would surprise the doctor more than the patient!

He noted that even terminal cases could be helped if the doctor did his very best and never lost sight of the fact that God sometimes works in mysterious ways.

Early graduates reported that this "never give up on your patient" attitude and a strong belief in the potential of results through Osteopathy helped them attain the results that practitioners with less faith had not achieved.

One graduate, Dr. Wilborn Deason, facetiously remarked later, "We just didn't know some of these conditions were incurable, so we went ahead and cured them anyway."

With the influx of students and the projection of many more in the future, the Old Doctor wondered if the new students could be exposed to the family atmosphere that had helped so many of the first class follow in his footsteps and model their own practice after his.

Andrew was also concerned about whether new faculty members, soon to be added to upgrade the curriculum, would be a problem since they were steeped in standard medical concepts. Would they be able to integrate the Osteopathic philosophy with their medical education in such a way that they could blend rather than produce conflict?

He had already had some problems with Dr. William Smith, an excellent anatomy teacher who on occasion had questioned some aspects of the Osteopathic concept. Would there be more such conflicts when there were more medical doctors on the teaching staff? Another potential problem was that his less educated early graduates would be teaching alongside doctors with degrees from prestigious medical colleges.

Even though these problems seemed imminent, Andrew had very little time to think of anything other than finishing the infirmary. Soon there would be even more patients and students to worry about. A new charter had been developed for the school.

On another front a real crisis was developing. There was an immediate need for legislation which would legitimize Osteopathy. Arthur Hildreth, a graduate of the first class, was assigned to work with the local county representative and district state senator and to inform them of this legislative need for Missouri.

Judge Ellison and a couple of young lawyers prepared the initial bill. The Old Doctor was not entirely pleased with it as it stood, but, they told him, it was a beginning. They had to start somewhere. After a few minor changes, the bill was finally presented in the House by Representative Grubb of Gibbs in Adair County and in the Senate by Senator Seaber of Kirksville. After a great deal more work, it was finally passed by both houses.

Dr. Hildreth, who had spent a great deal of time in Jefferson City and was looking forward to reporting a successful outcome, was shocked when Governor Stone failed to sign the bill. The implied threat of a veto finished any chances of getting legislation during that session of the legislature.

Returning to Kirksville, Arthur Hildreth felt sad about bringing home the bad news. However, the Old Doctor said he didn't feel too bad about its failure to pass. "We will have a much better bill next time and it will be passed," he said. He laughed and pointed out that there were still forty-eight state legislatures to work on before his "baby" would be legal.

The infirmary, with treatment rooms and a large lecture hall, was completed January 1, 1895. On the tenth of the month, the dedication ceremony was held with a large crowd in attendance, so large that more than three hundred people were unable to get into the memorial hall. The gathering included nearly all of Kirksville society with the exception of most of the M.D.'s and their wives. The mayor, city council, and other dignitaries sat on the rostrum for the program which lasted three hours. Thomas Still was commended for his design and for his work in speeding up the construction process. For two days following the evening ceremony, open houses were held for the many who had been unable to attend the formal dedication.

Andrew's office on the third floor was quite ornate, its walls lined with gifts from his students. Here he could stay away from the traffic always present near the treatment rooms. What impressed many visitors was the dissection room on the fourth floor where tables were set up for bodies that were to be dissected and studied. This room was popularly known as the "chamber of horrors." Since the profession had no legal status yet, the school soon found that there was a problem in obtaining cadavers.

During the time the building was under construction, many local citizens had thought Andrew was making a great mistake in building a structure the size of this "Temple of

Osteopathy." Dedication ceremonies were barely over when they saw that the number of patients being seen daily had doubled. It was apparent now that they had underestimated the amount of space needed.

People were arriving from all forty-eight states and several Canadian provinces. The prominent and wealthy were among the great number of patients waiting for treatment. This large number of people taxed space and personnel in efforts to meet the patient load. As a result, a hurry-up call was given to the contractor to add another forty feet to the building on the north side to accommodate patients as well as the students who were waiting to enroll.

In three short years, the growth of Andrew's institution was unbelievable and there was no indication this expansion would end soon. In this boom period, it was almost impossible for the administration to do any precise planning. The town of Kirksville was also having trouble in adding enough housing to accommodate the influx of students and patients. For a while, some were afraid this growth might slow down or even stop, leaving them with much unused space.

During the mid-1890s people were not in such a big hurry for results, so when they were told they must stay in Kirksville for two or three months they simply made arrangements to stay that long.

The charge for patient care was twenty-five dollars a month, which included three treatments a week. Though it was not recommended, a patient could be treated for only two weeks for fifteen dollars.

Sometimes all the space was filled with patients waiting their turn. Many were in wheelchairs and accompanied by helpers and there were many on crutches. This created a traffic jam in the hallway, so much so that patients found it difficult to get to the treatment rooms once their names were called. Although the staff tried to keep the halls free from congestion, it was difficult to accomplish with so many slow moving patients. Nevertheless, patients gave the staff considerable credit for keeping things moving so well with the great number of them being served.

There was a sense of destiny surrounding the operation of the institution. Faculty and students, as well as the people of Kirksville, felt they were a part of the development of a new science, and that they were building for the future. So they were willing to be a cog in creating a smoothly run operation.

It was indeed a thrilling period for everyone involved in Osteopathy. The exhilarating spirit touched nearly every resident of the town and they began to make their homes available for the tremendous inflow of patients. Some even added rooms to their houses for this purpose. Even more important to Andrew and his co-workers was the enthusiasm Kirksville residents showed for the development of his discovery.

There were, however, two groups in town that did not share in the exhilaration of this thrilling period of Osteopathy. One was the medical profession, which remained aloof. The other included saloonkeepers and stores that sold alcoholic beverages. The Old Doctor insisted that patients who consumed alcohol would not be welcome at his infirmary. If they expected to be served by the staff, they must absolutely abstain from hard liquor and beer.

The Old Doctor's system was now less than four years old. He was receiving prominent people from all over the country, and patients were coming from overseas as well. Rarely had a new profession become so successful in such a short time. All who were involved in the system knew that difficulties would arise, but they had faith they would be able to cope with whatever the future might have in store.

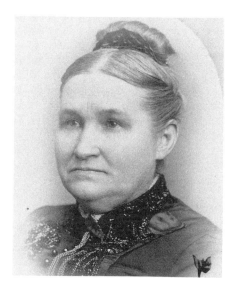

Mary Elvira Turner Still
("Mother Still")

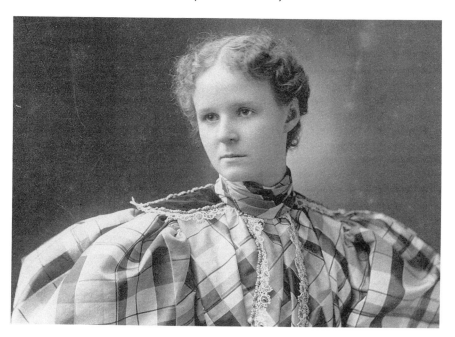

Blanche Still Laughlin
daughter of A. T. and Mary Elvira Still

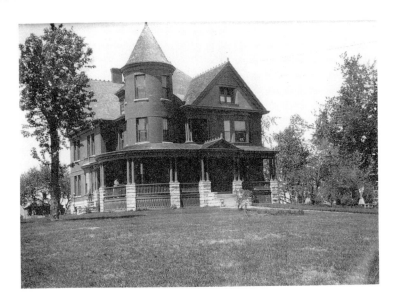

A. T. Still's Home in Kirksville about 1900

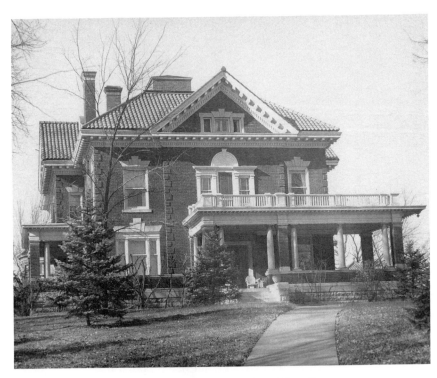

Charles Still's Home in Kirksville

Chapter Twelve

ARRY STILL FELT A BIT UNNERVED as he left the combined meeting of the School Administrators and Board of Directors. Thomas Still had shown the group his design for enlarging the Memorial Hall that at this point seated three hundred people. His plan would add space to the building along the north wall and adjacent to the current hall. By placing movable doors between the two halls, one thousand could be seated. This addition would also add more and crucial teaching space.

Harry had always been overly cautious in controlling the purse strings. By making such a demand for space, he felt that maybe their financial budget had been exceeded. It was quite possible that future growth would not justify such an expense.

However, he remembered that five or six years earlier he and other students had been crowded into a frame building designed to hold a mere seventeen students. If all of them showed up, there wasn't enough room to stretch their legs. He could remember his first anatomy class with the new faculty member, Dr. William Smith, a very tall man, even taller than Harry's father, Andrew. His wild hair was black, his slightly bulging eyes were black, and so was his shapely mustache. He exuded vitality and it would have been impossible to fall asleep during one of his classes. All the students enjoyed hearing him roll anatomical and medical terms around on his tongue, his Scottish accent giving a sort of musical quality. He had certainly been able to make anatomy real for his students, even before they had a dissection room. Harry had benefited from Smith's teaching. He knew he had learned a great deal.

He was aware of the problems his father had working with Dr. Smith because, except for their shared interest in medicine, they had very little in common. Dr. Smith was always looking for new challenges, and even with his great intellect it was hard for him to be highly successful in one position for a prolonged period. The Old Doctor found it difficult to understand the wanderlust which had taken Dr. Smith to several places and to many types of positions.

Dr. Smith was a fine lecturer, a qualified surgeon, and an excellent diagnostician. Yet, before he finished his first year at the school in Kirksville, he was already getting restless. Harry remembered when his father announced to the students that Dr. Smith had decided to take some time off from teaching in order to try his hand at practicing Osteopathy.

Even after Dr. Smith's departure, his influence was still present. During the last couple of months of the school's first year, Dr. Smith had taken under his wing one of the first women attending what was the very first class at the school, making her his number one assistant. This was Jeannette "Nettie" Bolles who was not only intelligent but was the first woman to receive a diploma from the school. She also proved, with additional help from Andrew, to be an excellent anatomy instructor.

Harry mused over how far the school had come in such a short period of time. He knew the family often spoke of him as the "family worrier." After the last planning meeting he realized that though he had always had his say in the past, the administration decided growth was essential and he thought he might as well let the other members of the board prevail – at least for the time being. He decided he could always take his money out of the operation later if he deemed the school was too risky a venture. He looked back on his success in establishing a lucrative practice in Minnesota and knew he could always fall back on that in case things did not go well in Kirksville. However, he was more than willing to do everything in his power to make his father's operation a success.

Harry was glad that his brother Charley and Henry Patterson, the school's secretary and business manager, had taken over the hiring and training of new faculty members. They had also done a first-rate job of supervising the growth of the clinical facilities and an infirmary staff that had the ability to handle the ever-growing patient load.

Even as the board was planning more growth, and with almost a dozen new faculty members on the staff, Osteopathy had not yet received its approval from the Missouri Legislature, which it was hoped, would pass a bill setting up Osteopathy as a separate profession and establishing its legitimate rights. This was a top priority, and Dr. Hildreth was once again spending much of his time in Jefferson City. This time he was talking to individual representatives. When he found one with a physical problem, he was happy to treat him gratis. While he was trying so hard to get an Osteopathic bill passed in Missouri, the home state of Osteopathy, the Vermont Legislature passed such a bill and became the first state to recognize this new profession. Vermont's action was soon followed by a bill approving Osteopathy in North Dakota.

With a new governor in office in Missouri, a revised bill was submitted by Judge Edward Higbee and presented to the Legislature. Because of Arthur Hildreth's work on it with the able assistance of Henry Patterson, the bill passed both houses and was immediately signed by Governor Lon Stephens on March 4, 1897. Osteopathy now had a law in its home state that allowed Osteopaths to practice legally on an equal basis with medical doctors.

It was a great victory, and there was much celebrating by Kirksville students and townspeople when the news arrived.

Medical opposition to this "upstart" profession, often bitter, for the most part had not been well-organized. Following this success, Dr. Hildreth moved quickly and almost single-handedly got a similar bill through the Michigan Legislature, which was signed by that state's governor shortly afterward.

The national medical organization decided that somewhere along the line it must make an organized stand if it were to stop the expansion of Osteopathy which was new competition for medical doctors. The group decided New York State should be the place to make a stand. So when new graduates were preparing to introduce a Practice Act before the New York Assembly in Albany, nearly all the "big guns" of the medical association were gathered in that capital city waiting to meet them head-on.

Dr. Hildreth, Patterson, and Harry and Charley Still were also in Albany and this time they were not feeling very confident about being able to pass their bill. Fortunately for them, the impending political battle received a lot of attention in New York City newspapers.

Mark Twain, the popular writer, had been treated by Andrew Still and other Osteopaths, as well. He had often enjoyed espousing the cause of underdogs and arrived in Albany in time for the hearings. He volunteered to help the Osteopaths in any way he could. There was an air of excitement in Albany when it was learned that the Osteopathic profession would have as one of its main speakers the noted writer and humorist, Mark Twain.

On the day of the meeting, the gallery was filled to overflowing, and when Mark Twain was introduced the gallery gave him a standing round of applause. This so incensed the medical group that one of them assailed Twain's qualifications. In addition, this spokesman characterized the humorist as a man whom no one took seriously. He also questioned whether Mark Twain had any attributes of common sense. This attack was followed by others. Three noted medical speakers took turns leveling blasts at the Osteopathic profession.

Twain carefully listened to the tirade of criticism and abuse against what he considered a Missouri profession and a worthwhile one at that. He had asked to be the first speaker for the D.O.'s.

When he was again introduced to speak, the humorist received another round of cheers from the gallery. Turning to the doctor who had been so critical of him, he bowed and said, "My general character was attacked a thousand times before you were born, sir. You have not succeeded in bringing to light more than half of my iniquities, for which I am thankful."

Twain continued to speak. "There are two great schools of physicians – doctors and grandmothers. The latter do more and know more than the former. It has been the proud boast of our republic that we have religious liberty and that we can choose our spiritual physician, as we like, to care for our soul's health. Why not allow the same liberty in caring for our bodies?" He indicated that he had faith in the new profession, and that everything he had heard against it sounded like persecution. He did this so eloquently that the assembly later passed the bill that was signed by the governor.

All these legislative successes and debates that occurred before the votes were cast emphasized the fact that the Osteopathic education needed upgrading and that this would have to be an ongoing process. Medical colleges were getting better; it would require an even greater effort from this new profession to be able to compete successfully in the future.

As more and more subjects were added to the school's curriculum and instructors to the school, the Old Doctor felt that time that should have been spent teaching the fundamentals of his science was being used instead to teach material of little use. The student should devote all his or her attention to mastering Osteopathic diagnosis and treatment.

Now there were state laws to comply with and requirements that often changed from year to year. Andrew knew that his school, the American School of Osteopathy (ASO), would have to add new courses to meet these regulations. His college, being the first, would have to strive to remain in the forefront of Osteopathic education.

There were already several new schools of Osteopathy in operation and some of them had become a problem for the profession. Quite a few lacked the financial structure to become first-rate institutions. Two or three even resembled second-rate schools and, even worse, some had tried to peddle Osteopathic diplomas in much the same way as the medical diploma mills.

From the beginning, ASO continued to improve its faculty and facilities. Already some students who had entered the other schools were coming to Kirksville because they felt they were not getting a good education elsewhere. They felt that unless they remedied this situation and studied at Andrew's school they would hardly be qualified to go into practice and be successful.

The Old Doctor, who had been through many other battles with the medical profession and had survived them to bring this new profession into existence, often said, "We need not fear our enemies who have contested every step we have taken. They can't harm us; their kicks are only a blessing in disguise. Our great danger, in fact the only danger that could threaten the future of Osteopathy, are the mistakes of those who profess to be our friends."

Even before the legislative success in New York, another important victory had been won in the adjacent state of Iowa. Yet many legislative battles were still to be fought before Osteopathy would have legitimate status in all forty-eight states. But that victory in New York was a guarantee of the eventual success of the profession.

With successful Osteopathic colleges operating in Des Moines, Kansas City, and Philadelphia, on the East and West Coasts, and in the South, there were now many graduates in practice all over the country. It was no longer necessary to go only to Kirksville for treatment. Even so, a large number of patients chose to go to the birthplace of Osteopathy. Many, in fact, hoped that the Old Doctor would see them in person. However, with such a dynamic growth of competition, the number of patients going for treatment in Kirksville was gradually decreasing. During this same period, however, more and more prospective students arrived, hoping to enroll at ASO.

An unexpected phenomenon developed. Many of the early graduates, after starting their practices in a particular town or city, began to feel that their locations "belonged" to them solely. They resented the arrival of other practitioners. It actually took several years before they found that additional members of their own profession in a community would be a help to them rather than a hindrance. As their practices expanded, these same graduates discovered there was no way any one person could take care of all the prospective patients in most communities, no matter how small a community. This was one of the first steps in creating a need for national and state organizations. The rapidly growing profession needed cooperation, not independent operators.

There were many changes taking place in Osteopathic education and practice. More and more courses were offered. With courses available in obstetrics, it was necessary to have a facility for the delivery of babies. When surgery was added to the curriculum, the need for a hospital became a high priority and one was built as soon as possible.

Andrew had been worrying about some of the new colleges that tried to get by on a shoestring and produced poorly trained graduates. However, there was nothing he could do to keep some unscrupulous individuals from starting colleges and calling them "Osteopathic." As the new association, representing the profession, was launched and grew, he hoped that it could do something to guarantee the quality of future Osteopathic graduates. The best he could do was to continually upgrade the faculty and facilities at his American School of Osteopathy.

Another college had opened in Kirksville as competition, and although it was at times a major annoyance, the ASO administration tried to exercise restraint in its relationship with it. At the same time, ASO continued its program of bettering its own institution.

With a faculty of twelve, two members holding medical degrees and one having a medical school education, it was a problem to keep the educational process moving smoothly. There was some resentment from Dr. William Smith who had returned to the faculty and the two Drs. Littlejohn over the fact that instructors with less education were being allowed the same authority in their teaching freedom and working for comparable pay. Dr. Charley, who had the title of vice president, but acted as the administrative head of the school, had to settle quite a few problems arising from this educational friction.

Dr. Charley also had another problem, one that was created by his father. Andrew was always a generous man. Knowing that the college was making money and that some students were financially strapped, Andrew told them that since they needed the money more than the school needed it, he would waive their tuition fee. So Charley often walked a tightrope as his job was to meet the payroll and at the same time keep the faculty and his brother Harry, who was treasurer, happy. Charley didn't want to question his father's authority, but he was responsible for meeting ongoing expenses.

He found himself in the position of contacting students who had benefited from his father's generosity and advising them that in some way or another a different arrangement would be required. He asked that they sign a note for a loan to be paid back later. If this information became public, it would make it most difficult for the school to collect fees from other students in the future. He had to do this in a diplomatic way so the new arrangement would not get back to his father.

In a short five years, the character of the student body had changed rather dramatically. During the first three years, nearly all of the students came from families whose members had benefited from Osteopathic services. Few of them knew whether a livelihood could be made from their new profession.

Now there were successful practitioners scattered all over the country, most of whom were doing quite well financially. There were now students enrolled at ASO who admitted they were there just to get a diploma and get out so they could go into the field and make money. In addition, the student body was not the closely knit family of the first few years.

There had also been changes in the town of Kirksville. With a population that had nearly doubled, there were many new stores, cafes, and transportation services. The grocery stores and restaurants had done a thriving business trying to keep up with the explosive growth.

Andrew was well aware of the benefits local people derived from the operation and expansion of the school and infirmary. He was more than a little miffed when several prominent businessmen financially backed Dr. Ward when he started a school in competition with ASO. Charley was not, however, a man to hold a grudge. In the past he had been the butt of ridicule by many who later came to him and apologized.

With the twentieth century approaching rapidly, the Old Doctor felt so surrounded by change that he decided it might be a good time to look back over the past decade.

IN REVIEW HE REMEMBERED that in 1890 the term "Osteopathy" – a word he just made up – had just been coined. As its originator, he was the only one then who had a complete understanding of this new therapeutic system – his system, his discovery. His sons had learned how to treat some conditions, but at that time they had very little knowledge of the total concept.

That was also true of the patients he had helped. They knew even less about how he had been able to help them. They were happy to have the benefits without trying to understand how the system worked. And at this time, he had been careful about discussing the details of his system.

While reminiscing, he could still painfully remember the rejections he had experienced earlier. He vividly remembered how, when he was developing his concept back in Kansas, Baker University had not allowed him to present his ideas on its campus even though his family had been involved with its founding. And he could not forget the preachers in Baldwin, Kansas and Macon, Missouri who had condemned his ideas as some form of witchcraft.

During all those early years when he was going from town to town as an itinerant doctor, he had usually either avoided or just touched on the concepts behind what he was trying to do. He had always been generous with his time, however, explaining to patients something about their condition and how he would be trying to help them. He had learned, though, that his discovery was simply too complicated for a public that thought that one must take a pill in order to expect a good result.

It was as an itinerant doctor that he had cast his lot with some of the quacks who went from town to town making wild claims that they could cure everything. And it was true that he was the subject of some of the same verbal abuse other itinerants received. But it was on these trips that he had been able to expand his skills. With his record of success, he had soon established such a sound reputation that, when the last decade of the nineteenth century arrived, and with his sons to train, he had decided to make Kirksville his base of operations and have his patients come to him.

HE CONTINUED TO THINK ABOUT the days before the infirmary when, during pleasant weather before the onset of winter, his patients gathered under the trees, often with picnic baskets, waiting to be seen. Many were lame and some were blind, but before he would treat any of them, he would go out on the lawn and join in their conversation. He enjoyed their laughter at some of his jokes. And he would often treat his patients right there under the trees. He hated to leave the outdoor atmosphere, but with so many more patients to see and the many months ahead of inclement weather common to northern Missouri, it had been imperative to move inside to year-round quarters.

It was important for the Old Doctor to remember that he felt in tune with the universe when he could be outdoors. Even when the weather chilled, he lingered outside under the trees. In this setting, he most likely did some of his best work. Certainly some of his deepest thoughts came into focus as he surrounded himself with nature.

He could remember agonizing over starting the school and naming this science. Would he actually be able to teach his science? His sons had been able to pick up some of the purely mechanical elements of his theory, but with their limited background, how could they ever grasp the principles involved? If it hadn't been for his children, he reflected, he would have avoided the headaches of starting his school.

Like so many others, he marveled at the explosive expansion of his system of therapy. He didn't have to look back any farther than a few short years to realize that, when he decided to make Kirksville his permanent home, if he was considered by the townspeople at all, they thought of him as a poor, wandering, unknown doctor with little influence and some very strange ideas about treating patients.

Even after some exceptional local successes, he had had a better reputation in some of the small surrounding communities than in his own hometown. The infirmary had been completed and large numbers of out-of-state patients were coming to see the Old Doctor before the local people used his services to any great extent.

He remembered that as the financial potential of his system began to be felt by local businesses, Kirksville had finally begun to take him seriously and had put out the welcome mat. He felt a degree of amusement when he recalled how many of the local people thought he had lost his mind when he built such a large infirmary and school complex. They had thought then it surely would end up as a white elephant. It was difficult for them to believe that it was outgrown before it was even completed.

He thought about how fortunate he was to have children who, most of the time, had been a real help to him over a long period. Again he thought about the lucky coincidence that had brought Dr. William Smith to him at exactly the right moment – the period when he was debating with himself about whether he should start a school.

Most of all, he kept thinking about how much of his success was due to the constant and loving support of his wife, Mary Elvira. She had so often cheered him on and had carried him through several financial crises. She always had faith in his ultimate success. He was extremely happy that "Mother Still," as the students called her, had been able to have a brand-new, rather large home built. He was also pleased that his daughter, Blanche, had become such a help to her mother. Sometimes he did think she was a little too bossy, especially when she sided with her mother to see that he cut down on some of his activities to preserve his strength.

He realized that teaching, seeing patients, and being involved in the operation of the school had used up more than their share of his energy. There were many days when he knew that he might be at risk from doing too much – but there was so much to be accomplished.

He had recently been persuaded to write his autobiography, which had taken a lot of his time and strength. Even before he had finished it he became painfully aware that he must get a book or two written on the practice of Osteopathy while he was able. So it was necessary that he begin to gather material and think it through so he would have a book of his own before too long that could be used by both students and graduates.

During the spring of 1897, many students who had finished in the early classes returned to the college for additional education. To meet changing requirements, these early graduates received this additional education from the school free of charge and were issued new diplomas which would comply with new state laws that had been enacted by several states.

It was these same early graduates who, while they were taking added classes, were insistent that the Old Doctor do as much writing as possible, particularly in the field of Osteopathic practice. He was quite pleased that these men and women, who, in most cases had developed successful practices of their own, were seeking him out to ask questions and to insist that he write books on the practice. They also urged him to get as many scientific articles on treatment, as often as possible, into the *Journal of Osteopathy,* which they found to be a very worthwhile magazine.

ANDREW WAS NOW SO BUSY that he tried to stay away from the problems of the school. But when some returnees, as well as some of the regular students, told him they were interested in obtaining an adequate number of cadavers, he remembered how helpful it had been for him to have an adequate number to study in order to get a firsthand knowledge of the human body.

He called in Dr. Smith and Dr. C. L. "Bob" Rider, his assistant, and asked them what the problem was. Dr. Smith explained there was no way they could compete with the established medical schools in procuring unclaimed bodies from state institutions such as prison and mental facilities. The state medical schools somehow or another had an inside track, it seemed. So far, the state of Missouri had no anatomical board to see that there was a fair and equal distribution of cadavers to the different colleges. At best, ASO received only a few when there was a surplus.

It was the fall of 1899 when, for some reason, the supply of cadavers had completely stopped. It was at a time when ASO needed them most. The majority of bodies available recently had come from poor farms. Now it seemed that ASO was always too late in bidding for the bodies.

ONE OF THE MORE COLORFUL incidents in the early history of Osteopathy resulted from this situation. Following is a summary of several versions reported on this affair.

One of Dr. Smith's anatomy students, a short time before the meeting the Old Doctor called about dissection, had told the teacher he had a relative on the Chicago police force who said one of the keepers of the Cook County morgue might sell several bodies at a price reasonable enough to make a trip to Chicago worthwhile.

Dr. Smith and Dr. Rider were eager to make the trip and bring back enough cadavers to enable the dissection room to operate at full capacity. They had a short talk with Dr. Charley. He told them that what they proposed was illegal and he felt the school shouldn't support such a venture.

Dr. Smith responded, "We really need the bodies and Bob and I are willing to take the risk." He said his students and the postgraduates needed all the bodies they could obtain to improve their understanding of anatomy. And with or without the school's approval, the two men said, they intended to go to Chicago.

As the two boarded the Burlington train to Chicago, they were assigned berth 13. Even though Dr. Smith was not superstitious, Dr. Rider said he hoped this was not a bad omen. When they were escorted to room 1313 in the hotel, Dr. Rider felt even more uneasy about their mission, although he kept these thoughts to himself.

Shortly after their arrival they contacted the police officer who was their liaison. He told them he would send around a Mr. Ullrich, the night watchman of the morgue, not the keeper. Since he was the only one on duty at night, this Mr. Ullrich would have access to the bodies and would not be questioned if any were missing.

Following their evening meal, Mr. Ullrich arrived at the hotel. He was not the type of person the doctors would normally associate with, but since they had been referred to him by the police officer, they felt it would be safe to do business with this unkempt person.

Mr. Ullrich said they should meet slightly after midnight. He said he would hire a driver and dray and bring along four boxlike trunks to pack the bodies for shipment. He told them the driver would require twenty dollars. The trunks would cost an additional sixty dollars, male bodies would cost fifty dollars each, and if female bodies were available, each would cost sixty dollars. He said he must have all the money in his hands before any bodies left the morgue.

The doctors put on their old clothes, packed four sheets to wrap the bodies, their embalming materials, and a large bottle of formaldehyde. Just before midnight, they headed for the Dunning Hospital and its morgue. Dr. Rider kept thinking, "This is still November thirteenth."

They boarded the last streetcar running that night and were let off at the end of the line, which was two miles from their destination. A misty rain and cold autumn wind swirled around them as they headed for the rendezvous, stumbling through the darkness. By the time they arrived, they were cold, wet, and muddy and wished the whole affair were over and they were safely home in Missouri.

The dray and driver were already at the front door of the morgue. The driver was as anxious as they were to be away from the unpleasant surroundings. The doctors quickly selected four bodies, three male and one female, and paid the night watchman. They were unpleasantly surprised when he told them they could not embalm the bodies in the morgue, but must move them out immediately. He said there was an old deserted house about a quarter-mile away that they could use for the embalming.

The driver of the dray was John Rowe, who seemed to be a nice person and helpful except when it came to moving the bodies. He simply would not touch them. So the doctors lugged out the four corpses themselves and loaded them onto the dray. The rain had increased and the night seemed even darker when they arrived at the empty house. There were no lights and the small candle they lit didn't help much as they tried to get embalming fluid into the veins. In such poor lighting, a procedure that should have taken an hour dragged on much longer. As they worked, the doctors got blood on their hands and clothes. There was no running water so it was impossible to clean themselves.

The driver was so anxious to leave that the two finally decided to wrap the bodies in the sheets and simply douse them with the formaldehyde to protect them for the train trip to Missouri. The corpses were at last packed into the boxes and addressed to Dr. Smith's home in Kirksville. They told Rowe to take the boxes to the American Express office at the

Burlington Station for shipment. Rowe said the boxes reeked of formaldehyde and they would probably have to be stored outdoors until the train left that evening.

The dray was quite a sight. Dr. Smith and the driver sat in front. Dr. Rider sat atop one of the coffinlike trunks. They finally arrived at the end of the two-mile ride from the morgue and Dr. Smith gave the driver an extra ten dollars. They both wished him well and watched him disappear into the misty wet night.

The hotel where they were staying was not close to the train station, so Rowe had suggested the doctors go back to the place where they had left the streetcar earlier. He thought they would get there about 5:00 A.M., about the time the first streetcar arrived. He said they would be more comfortable traveling back to the hotel in the streetcar since it was still raining.

It wasn't long before the streetcar arrived. The doctors were glad it was empty so no one would see their bloodstained clothes and disheveled condition. They picked up some old newspapers and sat on the back seat to shield themselves from view.

On the way downtown, the streetcar picked up very few passengers. However, several of them were policemen. Arriving at their stop, the doctors made a hurried exit, hoping the police hadn't noticed their appearance.

They made it to the safety of their room, took off their clothes, wrapped them in old newspapers, and packed them in their suitcases. They bathed and rested for several hours before dressing in clean clothing and going to a coffee shop for a late lunch. The train didn't leave until 8:00 P.M., so they had plenty of time to tour the city. Both felt relaxed and ready for a pleasant afternoon after the dreadful experiences of the previous night.

After ordering lunch, Dr. Smith bought an afternoon paper. They were shocked to read the headlines: "Body Snatchers Break Into Dunning Morgue and Steal Four Bodies." After their lunch arrived, they could hear other diners discussing the bizarre crime. Dr. Smith ate his lunch, but Dr. Rider was unable to eat a single bite.

They returned to their room to discuss the situation. Dr. Smith said he was puzzled. Why would Ullrich stage a robbery since he seemed to have such a good thing going. Since Ullrich and their police contact were the only ones who knew their identity, they felt safe wandering around Chicago. It was a good way to spend the warm afternoon.

However, their concern grew. The warm afternoon could create a problem since the trunks, reeking of formaldehyde, were sitting exposed to the heat on the station platform, with Dr. Smith's home address printed on them.

The late afternoon paper went into even greater detail concerning the robbery at the morgue. Already the superintendent of the morgue complex had offered a reward of five hundred dollars for information about the culprits – the two men who financed the venture and a dray driver. The story noted that all police in the city had been alerted to watch for suspicious persons who might have stolen the bodies.

The doctors cut short their walk through downtown Chicago and returned to their room where they stayed until time to catch the streetcar for Burlington Station. They even had their evening meal sent up to their room. When they arrived at the station, they checked to see if the trunks had been loaded. They were already in the express car and it seemed that no one had been suspicious.

As the train pulled out of Chicago, the two totally relaxed for the first time since the venture began. The bodies arrived safely in Kirksville and were in good condition.

For the first time in quite a while, Dr. Smith had enough cadavers to operate the dissection room. However, things in Chicago had really heated up. Ullrich had given the dray number to the police and John Rowe had been arrested while Ullrich had become eligible for the reward. The driver was so incensed for being turned in and charged with the crime that he refused to tell what he had done with the bodies. All he would say is that the other two men who were involved were from out of state and he did not know their names.

When the newspapers got wind of that, they really gave the police department fits. How, they asked, could two men from out of state come to Chicago, snatch four bodies, and safely move them through the city streets, probably shipping them by train to their home base, all without being apprehended?

With the uncooperative John Rowe in jail, and the city buzzing over this bizarre theft, an even larger reward was offered for information leading to the arrest of the two perpetrators.

Ullrich, who knew that Superintendent Healy wanted to replace him and had heard that a replacement had been found, saw an opportunity to cash in on the reward money. He had a prostitute friend go to the police and tell them that the night before the robbery she had met two out-of-staters and knew both their names and where they were from. For the reward, she would give the police the information.

When she told them the names and location of the two doctors, the city of Chicago was in such an uproar and wanting to bring the two criminals back that a special grand jury issued an indictment for the Drs. Smith and Rider. The city also urged the governor of Illinois to have them extradited.

After the governor of Missouri was notified, he asked the two doctors to meet him in Jefferson City. After all of the details of the events had been discussed, the governor, who had signed the Osteopathic law in Missouri, asked them why they had taken such a risk.

They reported how they needed cadavers for their dissection room and how hard it had become to obtain them. The governor said he would work out a way for them to get a fair share of corpses in the future. As far as the extradition request was concerned, he said, "Not a chance. If they got you over there, they would put you in jail for the rest of your lives."

Back in Chicago, the papers were screaming for the return of the doctors to stand trial for their "dastardly crime." In the meantime, Superintendent Healy, who had never trusted Ullrich, became suspicious that Ullrich had staged the break-in. He decided to investigate. After a short visit with John Rowe in jail, he was convinced that Rowe was telling the truth. There was no sign of a break-in at the morgue until after the dray and the bodies had left. When faced with this evidence, the prostitute admitted that she had never met the two doctors and that Ullrich had put her up to the whole thing so they could share the reward money. The superintendent was able to convince the police that the driver was innocent of any crime and should be released. Ullrich was soon charged with a variety of crimes.

Although Chicago papers still wanted the Missouri governor to turn the two doctors over to them for their part in the lurid event at Dunning, it wasn't long before they found material for new headlines to replace the morgue caper.

Chapter Thirteen

OR THE FIRST FIVE YEARS after Andrew gave his profession a name, business increased rapidly. Earlier, in 1895, when most patients were coming to Kirksville from only a three-state area Missouri, Iowa, and Illinois – and were inspired to come mostly by word of mouth, United States Senator Joseph P. Foraker of Ohio, a very prominent Republican, brought his ailing son to the Old Doctor. The child had not been helped by any of the nation's most outstanding medical centers that had treated him.

After only a few months of treatments in Kirksville, the boy made so much progress that his father suggested that Colonel A. L. Conger, chairman of the Republican National Committee, who had suffered a stroke, also visit Kirksville to see if the Old Doctor could help him. With both Foraker and Conger staying in town for several months, many other prominent political figures visited Kirksville to witness the wonderful improvements the colonel and the Foraker boy were making. The proof of what Osteopathy accomplished with these two helped spread the word of this new profession throughout the rest of the Nation.

Mrs. Foraker was so pleased with the recovery of her son that she bought a home in Kirksville in the summer of 1896 and lived there for another three years. She helped organize social activities for the local women and the women students. She was one of the organizers of the Sojourners Club, an organization that played a prominent role in local service activities. Anna Still, Blanche Still, and Judge Ellison's wife were charter members of the new women's club.

With all of the comings and goings of prominent Republican politicians, Andrew had the impression that it was at one of their meetings in Kirksville that they may have decided on William McKinley as their candidate for president in 1896.

There is no doubt that the senator and colonel were quite influential in telling the country about the marvelous cures the Old Doctor was achieving on a great variety of conditions. Earlier it had been a Presbyterian minister, the Reverend Mitchell, who had helped open doors locally.

Mrs. Conger was so impressed with what Osteopathy did for her husband that, a few years after his death, she enrolled in an Osteopathic college and was graduated.

When early ASO graduates returned for postgraduate training, they reported a growing organized opposition to the profession. National and state medical societies and some state boards of health were directing their efforts towards preventing any further growth of the Osteopathic profession in general as well as working against individual practitioners.

In defense, students decided to form an organization they hoped would give them leadership and support. The meeting to set up the new organization was held at the college on February 6, 1897, with four representatives from each class and a few recent graduates who lived nearby.

Six weeks later their draft was completed and sent out to fellow students, the school's graduates, and other colleges, inviting suggestions and cooperation. The original need for such an organization was to help graduates, especially those in states that had not yet enacted a practice act. In general, the organization was to do everything possible to legitimize Osteopathy. The name selected, American Association for the Advancement of Osteopathy, was soon shortened to American Osteopathic Association (AOA).

The association's first effort was primarily defensive and directed against organized medical opposition. After a meeting in 1901, however, emphasis shifted toward improving relations among Osteopathic colleges, standardizing educational requirements for Osteopathic curricula, and adopting a code of ethics that would improve relationships within the profession. It was also decided the association should publish a journal to represent all members of the profession. Arthur Evans was named editor and W. F. Link chosen chairman of the committee on publications. Since the two men lived in eastern Tennessee, Chattanooga was selected as headquarters for the new publication.

Earlier in May, 1894, a tabloid-size publication, *Journal of Osteopathy,* had been published in Kirksville. Most of the early editions reported on the Old Doctor's addresses, the school's articles of incorporation, and the successes of early graduates. The third edition carried a complete report on Dr. Charley's first year of practice in Minnesota.

By 1901, it was evident such a publication needed to appeal to graduates of the other Osteopathic colleges as well, so the first issue of the new magazine, published that September as the *AOA Journal,* was designed to fill that need.

Although the AOA organization had its roots in the ASO student body, after two years it was decided that only graduates of approved Osteopathic colleges could hold active membership. Fortunately for AOA and the Osteopathic profession, the association was blessed with officers who were knowledgeable, dedicated, and had an amazing insight into the future needs of their profession.

THE OLD DOCTOR had always tried to respect the opinions of his fellows and was rarely critical of an individual, even when one held views diametrically opposed to his. Nevertheless, Marcus Ward really put Andrew's love of humanity to the supreme test when he started the Columbia School of Osteopathy in Kirksville in 1897.

Many years earlier, before Andrew had opened his school, he had met Ward in Eldorado Springs, Missouri, where Ward was a patient. Ward had later followed Andrew to Kirksville for more treatment and often asked him to start a school so he could be in the first class. Ward was also the first nonfamily member to own stock in the company that operated Andrew's school.

After the school became so successful, some townspeople and Dr. Ward saw the financial potential of expanding Osteopathy. With their backing, the Columbia School of Osteopathy was founded. It soon became apparent that unless this new school used a variety of cutthroat tactics, it could not compete with Andrew's well-established ASO. As a result, representatives of the Columbia School began meeting trains to recruit prospective students, offering them an Osteopathic education at a much lower cost, free clinics, and other services, also free.

In the beginning of its operation, the ASO administration tried to ignore the competition and its tactics. Andrew was hurt that some businessmen in Kirksville, whom he had considered his friends, had jumped on board with a man like Ward simply to make money. Osteopathy, to Andrew, was a vehicle to serve mankind, not a money-making scheme.

It had become apparent that the new school and clinic, through its aggressive actions, was not interested in fair and open competition. The ASO administration decided to fight fire with fire, and became assiduously competitive in seeking students and patients.

Dr. Ward, who had continued his education at a medical school in Cincinnati, wanted his school to offer both M.D. and D.O. degrees. However, during the four years of its operation, the Columbia School lost so much money it ended up in bankruptcy.

It hadn't taken long for the town to grow tired of the bitterness and name-calling, so except for those who had supported Ward financially, everyone was glad to see the Columbia School close its doors. The American School of Osteopathy settled down to a normal operation in which the entire community could once again take pride.

Andrew had kept out of the bitterness until Ward claimed publicly that he was really the one who discovered Osteopathy. This was too much for the Old Doctor.

Andrew had a sudden urge to dig out his old army uniform that had been in mothballs for more than thirty-five years. He could tolerate a lot of abuse, he said, but for anyone else to claim the discovery of the science he had spent his whole lifetime developing – now that was real fighting talk!

Almost all the others in the Still family were as angered as Andrew over this incident. It took all of the tact and persuasion that Mother Still could employ to keep members of her family from going over and punching out Marcus Ward. If Harry hadn't been out of town during the time that Ward was most vocal in his claim to be the discoverer of Osteopathy, it is doubtful that even she would have been able to keep him from giving Ward a physical thrashing. Mother Still may have been the happiest member of the family on learning that the Columbia School of Osteopathy was closing and Dr. Marcus Ward was bidding farewell to Kirksville.

With the arrival of the twentieth century, there were not only great changes in the Osteopathic profession, but in the medical field in general. The allopathic profession had become dominant among the several existing schools of healing and was beginning to absorb the eclectic and homeopathic schools to form what was later referred to as the "regular" school of medicine. Although not well respected by the medical profession at that time, pharmacology was developing into a science and researchers were beginning to study the effect of medication on the human body.

The American Medical Association (AMA) had now begun to weed out fly-by-night and second-rate medical schools and unqualified doctors within its own ranks. It was only the beginning of a trend, but it certainly indicated that medical leaders intended to upgrade their profession. There were, however, quite a few medical planners unsure of the best way to accomplish this goal. Also, there was no consensus on how to handle the upstart osteopathic profession.

Some medical doctors had noticed that when they were too bitter in their attacks, the public became sympathetic to the Osteopaths and it was easier for their competitors to pass laws giving them legal rights to practice. This had proven to be true on an individual basis. When medical doctors were too vocal in criticizing new Osteopaths who entered practice, they often found that their remarks became a pat on the back, rather than a kick in the pants.

Some medical leaders suggested that if this upstart profession were left alone, it might destroy itself. There were others who hadn't fared too well in head-to-head competition with Osteopaths. Many of those swore they would torpedo this Osteopathic ship before it went much further.

Meanwhile, in the Osteopathic camp there was also a division of thinking regarding what courses should be added to the curriculum. One school of thought was that if too many medical subjects were added, it would weaken the emphasis placed on the Osteopathic concept. Others felt that to compete in the future with better-trained medical doctors, they must have a total medical education, including the proper use of proven drugs.

This was a problem that was to continue in spite of Andrew's opposition to adding courses in drug therapy to his school. Another emerging problem, present in many colleges, was the inability of faculty members to get along with each other, but such petty jealousies were accentuated at ASO because of the great divergence of educational backgrounds among the faculty.

This situation came to a head when Dr. Hildreth, who had received only a high school education plus training at ASO, was appointed as dean. This appointment caused quite a rebellion among the medically trained faculty members even though Andrew and most of the other faculty members supported Hildreth. This event brought the debate about the curriculum to a head.

Dr. Smith, who had been such an important figure in the development of the profession, decided to resign after leading an unsuccessful revolt against Dr. Hildreth's appointment. By now the school had nearly twenty faculty members and seven hundred students. Everyone felt sorry over the loss of this great anatomy teacher, but Dr. Smith had set such a high standard of excellence that, even with his departure, his department continued its level of quality education under Dr. Will Laughlin, who took over the program.

As the background of the faculty grew more diverse, newer members sometimes criticized the behavior of the Old Doctor. If anything, he had become even sloppier in the casual attire he had always worn. And his habit of wandering in and out of classrooms became quite annoying. Even though he wore boots, he was so quiet that the teacher would only discover his presence when the students began to stare in Andrew's direction. Sometimes, he would stay for only a few minutes and then disappear as suddenly as he had arrived. On other occasions, he would take over the lecture and then leave without paying specific attention to the professor. This was quite disturbing to the teachers, but they felt they could not complain about the founder's behavior, certainly not to him, and to call attention to their feelings would accomplish nothing, they realized.

One day, Andrew strode into a classroom, took up a piece of chalk and told the class he was going to draw a pig. He started drawing what slightly resembled a pig and as he blocked out the students' view with his body, added some feathers. His picture ended up looking like a turkey.

He turned to the class and asked, "How do you like my pig?"

Many admitted it wasn't too bad. But as he moved away, he showed the changes in his drawing.

"Be sure," he said. "Just because someone says something is so, don't take their word for it. Make your own decisions and find out for yourself or you may end up being the turkey!"

He added, "Don't trust anyone completely, not even this Old Doctor."

He continued visiting classrooms and always stressed the importance of discovering for oneself the underlying cause of any abnormal condition.

With his reduced teaching load, Andrew had more time to devote to other areas that interested him. As deeply involved as he was in the development and growth of his profession, the Old Doctor never lost interest in other happenings in the world. He maintained his interest in plant and animal life. He took time to study rocks and geological formations and the movements of the stars. He also had some inventions he felt he should develop. Politics and social trends captured his attention, too.

One popular interest at this time throughout the Midwest was called spiritualism. Nearly every town of any size had a group meeting regularly to discuss this topic. Many people believed that the Old Doctor, because of his intuitive approach to diagnosis, had special powers. With his wide range of interests, Andrew attended the local and statewide spiritualists' meetings for a short time.

Some of the new faculty were upset by Andrew's involvement in spiritualism and claimed they were embarrassed that the head of their institution would attend meetings of such an unscientific "fringe" group. For a long time, Andrew paid no attention to their criticism. He remarked that "no one should look down on something they don't understand" and that was one reason he was trying to stay informed of any ideas that might be of value.

Finally, after one faculty member came to him and said he and his colleagues didn't think it was appropriate for the president of the college to be seen attending such an unscientific group, Andrew called the faculty together. He asked them what they did in their spare time. Several reported they played cards or attended dog shows or horse races. Others said they attended a variety of other sporting events. The Old Doctor suggested, then, that it was possible he had expanded his overall knowledge more by what he was doing than they had by playing cards, attending dog shows, or other sporting events, and this quieted faculty criticism for a time.

In spite of the occasional criticism of his outside activities, nearly all new faculty members were deeply interested in learning all they could from him while they were earning their D.O. degree. This was just as true of the rest of the faculty.

Though there was firsthand exposure to the teachings of the founder and to the zeal he instilled in his students, there was a great turnover. Many wanted to go into practice as soon as possible. There were also quite a few changes in the faculty, in the administration, and in the front office.

Henry Patterson, the business manager who had served the school with distinction, and his wife Alice, left to pursue a practice in the nation's capital. George Laughlin, who had married Blanche Still, had a Master's degree along with his

D.O. He became dean. Warren Hamilton was now business manager. Shortly after taking this post, Hamilton became one of the first outside the Still family (besides Dr. Ward) to own much stock in the company that operated the school, infirmary, and hospital.

Another challenge about the operation of a college that this century presented was student behavior in general and drinking alcohol in particular. During the first few years he operated the school and infirmary, the Old Doctor's mandate against the use of alcohol by patients, students, and faculty had been generally observed by the student body. But within the first five years of the new century, much of the close family atmosphere that had so characterized the operation of the institution in the 1890s began to disappear.

Dr. Ward, in the four years that he operated the Columbia School of Osteopathy in Kirksville, never imposed any restrictions on his students. Now with the large number of new students – men and women – coming into town to attend ASO, it became increasingly difficult to maintain the school's prohibition of alcohol consumption.

A few years later, after the development of fraternities and sororities, the Old Doctor was aghast to find that their parties involved consuming not only beer, but hard liquor. This came to his attention one Saturday afternoon when he saw a strange flag flying over one of the fraternity houses. On a large white background, there were large blue letters that spelled out "Sunny Brook Cruise," the name of a whiskey. He seriously considered banishing the fraternal organizations, but after they agreed to refrain from such activities, Andrew relented and allowed them to continue their existence.

A continuing concern was the school's relationship with the townspeople and officials of Kirksville. In the past there had been a great worry that Andrew would move the college to a larger city. However, he and his college had stayed in

Kirksville and time had proved that his loyalty to the town was unshaken. To assuage such concerns further, if they still existed, in October of 1900 Andrew sponsored a picnic for all the residents of his hometown and for everyone in Adair County, honoring residents and his student body.

Everyone was given a tour of the school and its facilities, followed by a parade with a band and several marching units. The event was such a success that it was repeated the following year when townspeople called it the "Andrew Still Day," giving schoolchildren a half-day holiday.

The school administrators were particularly interested in having the students and townspeople become better acquainted for a variety of reasons. One was that students had so organized their classes that class rivalry sometimes spilled over into some free-for-alls, using the town square as the site for some rather active fracases. Another reason was that fraternity hazing had involved the local fire department that had been called to rescue students who had been required to climb to the top of the water tower at the railroad station and hadn't been able to get back down. Another was that the mayor of Kirksville had often been asked by Dr. Charley to get some of the more boisterous students out of the local jail.

So, for these reasons, as well as Andrew's fierce loyalty to and appreciation of his hometown, the picnic and the celebration of the Andrew Still Day gave the townspeople a chance to see that students could behave themselves and be first-class hosts.

During this same period, Osteopathy was continuing to grow in popularity across the nation and around the world. Although the number of patients coming to Kirksville for treatment was slowly decreasing, there were still enough people arriving to tax all available housing facilities. There were more and more affluent patients. Some even lived in private railroad cars parked on a side track near the station.

Because of their wealth and position, many wanted to be seen by the Old Doctor himself. However, Andrew was more interested in the most challenging cases, and since he wasn't impressed by wealth he often let the wealthy sit and wait their turn. Seeing Andrew in his sloppy dress, a few wealthy patients thought he was the janitor and chose to be treated by his better-dressed assistants.

This amused Andrew. But it was a way to get rid of some of his work load. He was also amused by patients who got off the morning train and demanded a cure in one treatment, no matter how chronic their condition might be, so they could return home on the afternoon train.

Andrew's sense of humor had carried him through some rough periods. One of his great charms was the fact that he enjoyed not only playing jokes on other people, but having jokes played on him. This brought him even closer to the students, who from time to time planned some harmless prank involving the Old Doctor. About the only thing that Andrew would not tolerate in these pranks was anything that might put his profession in a bad light. Otherwise, he was always a good sport.

He was also known for his tolerance toward his students. He enjoyed advising them, particularly when they first arrived to work in the clinic. However, after they had worked in the infirmary for a while, he became more demanding regarding their work. If they continued to give only routine treatment that the Old Doctor called "engine wiping," he became furious and told them that if they couldn't find the source of the problem they shouldn't plan on graduating.

He often repeated his belief that if there was an abnormal condition it was essential to find the problem, fix it, and then leave it alone. He couldn't tolerate mindless routine manipulative procedures. On one occasion his eldest son, Dr. Charley, had given a treatment to an overweight woman. The whole treatment appeared superficial to Andrew. It seemed to him that Dr. Charley had made no attempt to reach the cause of her problem. Andrew suggested in no uncertain terms that "promiscuous pummeling" would be of little value to this patient or to any other patient.

Over the years, Andrew had developed such a fine-tuned sense of touch, such an ability to perceive even the slightest deviation from the normal, and yet be able to put all of this into perspective in his consideration of the body as a complete unit, that there were still those who believed he was intuitive and that his considerable skill at physical diagnosis could not be taught to others. It may be true that no one ever reached Andrew's level of achievement at finding and correcting physical problems. However, there were many of his graduates who also developed a great ability in physical diagnosis and corrective manipulative procedures.

As skilled as the Old Doctor was in physical diagnosis, he was happy to learn of Roentgen's discovery of the X ray and recognized that soon there would be an additional aid to visualizing structural problems. His school was the second institution west of the Mississippi River to purchase one of the new X-ray machines. The newly formed X-ray Department with the new equipment was placed in the capable hands of Dr. David Littlejohn, the youngest of three brothers who had come from Scotland to teach at ASO.

In his own practice, Andrew had always stressed the positive. Although he knew that some cases were terminal conditions, he felt that failure only existed when a doctor accepted defeat without giving even the most unfavorable appearing case every opportunity to improve, or even to recover.

Many of his graduates followed his example and proved that careful manipulation, after establishing a correct diagnosis, produced success, not some special power that only the Old Doctor possessed.

By 1902, with nearly twelve hundred ASO graduates in the field, the *Journal of Osteopathy* began documenting the successful management and good results obtained by Osteopathic treatment for a great variety of diseases and physical abnormalities. By then, the *AOA Journal* was publishing the writings of men like Charles Hazzard and Carl McConnell. These men and others clearly had the ability to make the principles of Osteopathy more accessible to the public. Andrew's style of writing and his rather constant use of allegorical references made it difficult for some readers to be certain of his meaning. However, with so many well-trained writers now carefully describing the basic elements of the Osteopathic concept, the public was better informed.

As valuable as the writings of other Osteopathic teachers were in making this new science easier to understand, it often took the Old Doctor, speaking in parables and using strange allegorical situations in his lectures, to prove his point, though it was often obscure. This captured the attention of his students and made many of them strain their mental capacities to understand.

He often pointed out that "man comes into the world as a mental blank and even after a so-called 'education,' could leave the world in the same condition." Many educators teach only how to be good imitators and follow in the rut of popular thinking. But to his classes, Andrew stressed how necessary it was for the students, in their new profession, to develop their creative thinking so the full potential of their practice could be realized.

He often discussed his theories about living. He ended many of his presentations with the advice that "the Great Architect of the Universe," as he referred to God, "brought us into the world to help Him build an even better world. Listen, learn, and know thyself. And be at peace with God."

Many lectures of this dedicated, vital, and sincere man were followed by thunderous applause from his students. This might be considered somewhat unusual by present-day students, but it was common at the close of the Old Doctor's lectures.

Andrew was now approaching his midseventies. In spite of that, he maintained much of his vitality, appearing to be a tall and sturdy man. He wore a heavy blue serge suit, winter and summer, with a cap pulled down over his forehead, a wool muffler tied around his neck throughout the school year, and the usual boots on his feet. In his hands was a solid hickory staff that he would carve with his penknife from time to time. The markings were a variety of symbols that he often added to or changed entirely.

In spite of his unpleasant experiences with organized religion, based on what was judged as his "strange behavior," Andrew was a most religious man. He rarely failed to give the Creator full credit for his many successes, and admitted that "only by working through nature and the Creator can the great expectations of life be attained." He never felt it was necessary for him to attend church to further his religious life and did not urge his wife or children to attend. On the other hand, he never criticized the church affiliations they chose for themselves. As a result, many of his immediate family became members of the Methodist Church, notwithstanding the problems Andrew had experienced because of the behavior of Methodist preachers earlier in his career.

June 5/02.

Dear Dr. Still:

I remember you very well, & I wish I could accept your kind invitation, but my time is filled up & I am obliged to deny myself the pleasure.

Truly Yours

SL. Clemens

Letter of Samuel Clemens to A. T. Still

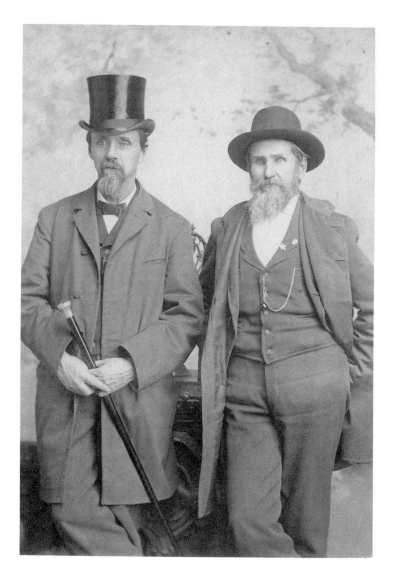

A. T. Still and his brother Edward

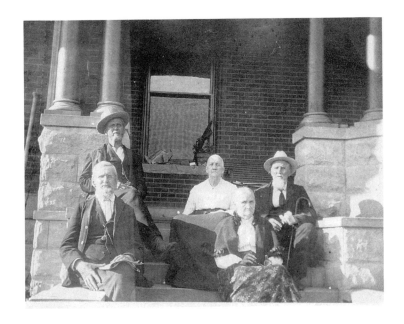

Members of the Still Family
back row, *l.* to *r.:* Andrew T. Still, Rahab Still, James M. Still
front row, *l.* to *r.* Edward C. Still, Mary Elvira Still

Chapter Fourteen

ROM THE TIME ANDREW began to develop the mechanical principles leading to the establishment of the science of Osteopathy, he concentrated on studying all aspects of the function and anatomy of the human body. He treated all kinds of diseases and physical abnormalities. His skill at reducing injuries and providing rapid relief for strains and dislocations, injuries that occurred so often on the frontier, earned him early recognition. Until the early 1870s, most of these injuries were farm-related or caused by falls around the house or barn. About the only sports-related injuries he treated were from hunting accidents. Perhaps an eager or sleepy hunter fell out of a tree while waiting for deer or other game to appear.

Although baseball is reputed to have been created in 1839 in Cooperstown, New York, many of its rules were not developed until 1845 by Alexander Cartwright. Until the Civil War, baseball was played primarily in the East, but this changed soon after the war because many of the farm and city boys from all over the country had learned the game during their army stints. Within a few years, nearly every town of any size had its own baseball team. Pitchers and catchers were usually paid and in many cases represented several different town teams in a short period of time.

With Andrew's reputation as a "lightning bonesetter" whose treatments proved to be so successful, many injured athletes came to Kirksville to be treated by him. Thus he became known as a pioneer in sports medicine.

By 1876, the National Baseball League had been formed. Andrew was seeing more and more baseball players with many types of traumatic conditions. However great his previous successes, he was disappointed that he couldn't help his son. Charley, home on furlough from Fort Leavenworth, wanted his father to correct his pitching arm injured during a game for his army team. After careful examination, Andrew told Charley there was probably a tear of the supportive soft tissue (perhaps a rotator cuff), and the problem could not be fixed by manipulation.

Football, like baseball, started in the East. In the beginning, it was probably a modification of rugby. In 1878, the University of Michigan was the first school to take the game west. Its team competed with Canadian schools, playing by Canadian rules, for the next few years. Over a period of fifteen years, the game began to resemble football that was played during the early decades of the twentieth century.

Midwestern colleges followed a variety of rules when they first played the game; some played four twelve-minute innings rather than quarters, some played without time-outs, and some played with more than eleven men on each side. This created a need to standardize the rules about 1889.

During the last decade of the nineteenth century football, like baseball, spread through the Midwest. It, too, was played by colleges as well as by town teams and high schools. The physical violence of this new sport brought a new variety of athletic injuries. Around Kirksville, many of the worst cases were brought to Andrew because of his reputation as an excellent diagnostician and manipulator. Although it was many years before this became a specialty, what Andrew was doing was pioneer work in the field of sports medicine – a field in which D.O.'s can now become certified.

Andrew had learned to understand baseball when he followed his son's baseball career in the army. He had been thrilled by the Fort Leavenworth victories over Fort Riley with his son on the mound. But football, unlike baseball, proved to be a game the Old Doctor couldn't understand. He could not figure out why men would risk their bodies in a game so conducive to injuries.

The Old Doctor had been so busy during the first few years of operating the school and infirmary that he had had little time to think about the development of sports or how sports-related injuries would involve Osteopathy.

Many students enrolling at ASO in the last half decade of the century had backgrounds in sports. Most athletic competition at the school was interclass baseball and football. Students formed a baseball team and played against town teams. During the fall of 1899, with the approval of the administration, students formed a football team and played seven games without a coach. The competition that year consisted of games against four town teams and two small college teams. The ASO team won three games and lost four. They played one town team twice and lost both times. Andrew regularly attended athletic events when they were held in Kirksville, and even though he never understood football he was always present to give support to "his children."

Dr. Charley and the administration were strong supporters of expanding ASO's participation in college sports. By the fall of 1900 they hired Ernest White, a full-time experienced football coach from the University of Missouri. The school also began construction of an athletic field to be completed by the 1901 season.

The Old Doctor, always a strong competitor, felt the competition his students faced on the athletic field would help prepare them for the stresses of starting practice in a none-too-friendly world. Even though he grew up in an era when few people had time for sports, Andrew realized students needed exercise to stay in shape, and he gave his full support to he recommended that a great variety of athletic competitions be made available and that the students be encouraged to participate.

The Still Athletic Field had its grandstand in one corner of the playing field, making it ideal for baseball. Temporary seats were set up for the football field, with a plan to put in permanent seats as the football program expanded and more seating was required.

The first football season under an experienced coach was a good one for the Osteopaths, as they called the team. Following a bitter loss to the University of Missouri Tigers in the first game of the season, the team won seven games, losing only one more.

When the 1901 season opened, students, faculty, and townspeople were excited. With an outstanding coach, some excellent players, and an expanded schedule, they looked forward to competition against some outstanding college teams.

The first two games were at home against teams that were not too strong and ASO's Osteopaths defeated them without problems. The third game was in Lincoln, Nebraska against a strong Cornhusker team. Although the Osteopaths played well, they finally lost in a close 5-0 contest. After this excellent showing against the fine Cornhuskers, the town was buzzing as the ASO team prepared to return to Columbia to see if they could avenge the loss of the year before.

Nearly everyone remembered how the team and its fans had been treated on the last visit to Columbia. Fans had been mauled by an unruly group of Missouri Tiger supporters. A real embarrassment to the ASO team grew out of an incident when Tiger fans tore the Osteopaths' colors off the special train and provoked ASO students and Osteopath fans. When a few fights broke out, several students and a couple of faculty members, as well as Dr. Harry Still, were hauled off to the Columbia jail and charged with unruly conduct and fighting.

When the ASO team prepared to invade Columbia again, nearly every able-bodied man in Kirksville had been recruited and boarded the special train, and Coach White was pleased to see so many in the stands wearing the red and black colors of his team. The coach was happy with the way his team completely outplayed the Tigers and handed them a 22-5 defeat. This time there were no problems as fans and players made a triumphant trip back to their hometown.

During the early years of football, eligibility rules were almost nonexistent. It was not unusual for a college to pick up players who weren't attending their school and probably weren't even living in the community. These "ringers" or "tramp athletes" were still playing for colleges in fairly large numbers at the beginning of the twentieth century.

The situation at ASO was considerably different. Some of its players had played at other colleges, but many were tired of going from one school to another just to play football. They wanted a profession instead, one that would offer a good financial potential.

Some outstanding athletes came to Kirksville with athletic injuries and after their recovery enrolled at the college. These additional and talented players helped make the 1901 team quite a powerhouse.

Although the school was less than ten years old and organized sports only in the third year, the ASO team played 13 games, scoring 379 points, while their opponents scored only 65. With wins over the University of Missouri, the University of Texas, and the Missouri School of Mines, and a 5-point loss to Nebraska and an 11-point loss to the University of Kansas, the Osteopaths emerged as a formidable football team. Unfortunately, this created a problem. Smaller colleges no longer wanted to play against a team with so much talent and larger universities didn't want to risk a loss to a small school like ASO.

With the athletic field completed, everyone looked forward to the 1902 season. Most of the better players on the team were still available, but Coach White had retired and the University of Illinois was the only major college in the football schedule. ASO's hopes took a downturn. This was not helped when several games scheduled for ASO's home field were canceled, some with less than a week's notice. Thus, the administration began to rethink its ideas about expanding its athletic program, especially football. In the end, it was decided to give it another try.

For the 1903 season, the administration hired a coach who was already a football legend, Pat O'Dea, an Australian by birth. He was a University of Wisconsin first all-American. He had gained fame as the greatest dropkicker in American football and was often referred to as "the human kangaroo."

On occasion he demonstrated his skill by drop-kicking a ball sixty-five yards or more with great accuracy. In 1899, before the Wisconsin-Yale game in New Haven, Connecticut, he gave a demonstration of both drop-kicking and punting that earned him national coverage and, shortly afterwards, was invited to become the head coach at Notre Dame.

With O'Dea as coach, ASO was able to schedule games with the University of Illinois, University of Wisconsin, and Notre Dame for the 1903 season. Unfortunately for hometown fans, these games were played on the road. Several times during this season there were again some last-minute cancellations.

The team played well, although it lost all three of its games against strong major colleges. Even before the team entrained for South Bend to meet Notre Dame, a decision had been made to de-emphasize football at ASO. In spite of its famous football figure to head the program, it was obvious that Kirksville was hardly the place to try to compete with major colleges that were then making football the hub of their sports programs.

major colleges that were then making football the hub of their sports programs.

After an all-night train ride, the Osteopaths played well against the undefeated Notre Dame (no team had even scored on the Irish that year). The team also had the opportunity to play against a Notre Dame legend, all-American Louis "Red" Salmon, a player who scored thirty-six touchdowns during his career at South Bend.

Even though they lost to the outstanding Notre Dame team by a score of 28-0, they impressed representatives of Madison Square Garden in New York who were considering a postseason round-robin competition, and the team later received an invitation to play in the New York event during the holidays. However, the promoters were unable to complete the necessary arrangements and the plan was abandoned. (Post-season games had not yet caught on. The first Rose Bowl game had been played in only 1902, and it would be fourteen more years before the second Rose Bowl game would be held.) Nonetheless, the value of athletic competition was quite obvious to the ASO administration. Not only did it help the students improve their physical condition, but the related injuries gave them a chance to see and treat a variety of conditions.

Because the school now decided to put less of its budget into competing with major football powers, additional funds were available to support other sports programs such as increasing the number of students involved in intercollegiate and interclass athletics.

It had been easy to bring both baseball and track teams from other colleges to Kirksville to compete on a "home and home" basis. This meant alternating home field advantage to provide fair competition. The administration felt that as soon as the de-emphasis on football had been completed, it would once again be able to bring small college football teams back to their home field.

ing that some became team doctors for college and town teams. In addition, many who entered practice in small towns became the team doctor for the local high schools. This activity gave them contacts that often helped them become family doctors, as well.

One of the problems that faced the administration when they considered de-emphasizing football was the rather large, two-year contract they had offered Pat O'Dea to come to Kirksville. This difficulty was solved, however, in a rather strange and mysterious way. After the last game that ASO was ever to play against a major college team, the Notre Dame game on November 7, 1903, Coach O'Dea disappeared. He was not heard of again for many years. There were many conflicting rumors as to what actually happened. According to a University of Wisconsin athletic department report, O'Dea moved to a small town in northern California and changed his name to Charles Mitchell. The report further stated that he was tired of football and its attendant fame. The only thing that is certain, however, is that some forty years after his mysterious disappearance, he attended a football game on the Stanford University campus and briefly talked to the press. He did not volunteer any details of why he had disappeared or where he had spent the intervening time.

Another strange twist to this mystery is that, even though he had served as track and football coach for Notre Dame during 1900 and 1901 and had led the team to its first football championship (with a two-year record of fifteen wins and four losses), there is very little written about him in the Notre Dame sports archives even though other coaches, with lesser accomplishments, received more attention.

There also seems to be no explanation why O'Dea had left a better-paying job at Notre Dame and taken a lesser-paying, less prestigious position at the University of Missouri. The one thing that is clear is that he never returned to Kirksville to receive his pay for the last year of his contract with ASO. Pat O'Dea was one of the early "greats" of American college football and his mysterious career remains an enigma to this day.

The last year that ASO played football with a paid coach was 1904, but the team still had talented athletes and again played against teams with less talent. Also, there were last-minute cancellations which left them playing against only five teams that year. Even though the team was undefeated, it was difficult to call it a successful season.

Football wasn't played again until the 1907 season. With a student as coach, the team was in a position to play small schools without the concern about last-minute cancellations. During the period in which there was so little football competition on the Still Athletic Field, more and more fans were attending intercollegiate baseball and track competitions.

The Old Doctor loved baseball and he always stayed until the last out. He was thrilled one year when his "boys" beat the University of Kansas in an extra-inning contest.

The athletic field was in almost constant use. Of all the sports in the spring, the highlight of the season was the annual baseball game between the talented ASO team and the faculty. Many of the team's former players worked in the clinic or taught, so it was often an exciting and close game. It was a good way to end the baseball season. It also gave Dr. Charley an opportunity to stand on the mound once again and throw a few pitches before his replacement took over. He would demonstrate the grip of his famous curve ball to the other pitchers.

College baseball teams continued to come to Kirksville to compete for a number of years, bringing a good level of baseball to the Still Athletic Field. In football, ASO had only competed three years against major universities, but in baseball this continued a few years longer.

With the combination of an excellent background in anatomy and skill in manipulation, it is not surprising that many ASO graduates turned their skills to the field of sports medicine. Among them were men like Wilbur Bohm. He was a track star who entered the Olympic tryouts in both the discus and shotput and later served both college and professional teams. Harrison Weaver, another ASO graduate, ministered to the Saint Louis Cardinals baseball team for twenty-eight years and also developed some improvements in athletic equipment that have proven quite useful. These are but two of the many ASO graduates who dedicated their lives to the ever-expanding need for treatment of sports injuries. Probably the best-known sports figure who ever attended ASO was Forrest "Phog" Allen, the illustrious coach whose teams won 771 basketball games during his long career at the University of Kansas.

Basketball came comparatively late to ASO. It was 1915 before a dozen interested former high school and college players organized a team without a coach. This "team" drove two old cars through the southern states, playing smaller college teams along the way, returning to Kirksville with a winning record.

Over the years many Osteopathic students competed in sports and treated athletic injuries. This emphasis and exposure helped the Osteopathic profession in pioneering sports medicine and in creating the momentum that caused this specialty to expand and be innovative even up to the present time.

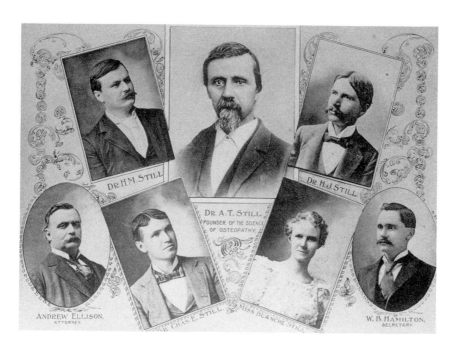

Early Board of the A.S.O.

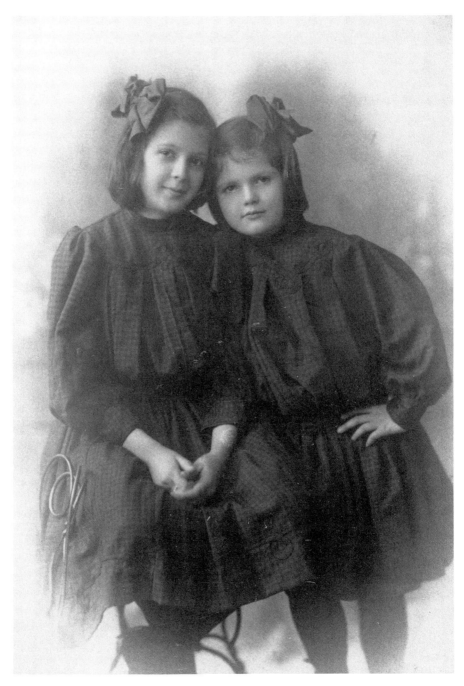

Gladys and Elizabeth Still

Chapter Fifteen

URING THE EARLY YEARS of the twentieth century, the growth of the school continued phenomenally, requiring a corresponding enlargement of faculty and need for more clinical facilities. A concern of the administration was the high turnover of its faculty. After receiving their degrees and participating in short teaching terms, many decided to practice Osteopathy for the experience and potentially greater financial rewards. There were some who really liked teaching and stayed on, fortunately, so that there was always a nucleus of qualified instructors at ASO.

Extended family members were also attracted to Kirksville to study Osteopathy and several stayed after graduation to become faculty members. These included Andrew's brothers Ed, Jim, and Thomas, the latter from California. Also, Mary Elvira's three nephews Guy, Mack, and Turner Hulett from Kansas. And his son-in-law's brother, Will Laughlin. Several left after a while to go into private practice. But three, Guy and Mack Hulett and Will Laughlin, stayed to become outstanding faculty members and Ed Still became a member of the clinical staff.

Andrew's son Herman had moved to Texas after pioneering Osteopathy in Illinois. Harry again desired to go back into practice and in 1903 sold his stock in the school to his brother, Charley, and Warren Hamilton, the school's business manager. Herman left for Chicago where he soon established a very successful practice.

217

The financial position of the school continued to improve and its stock began paying substantial dividends. Indeed the returns were so good that Mother Still was finally able to have her new home properly furnished without worrying about the cost.

Charley had had a lifelong interest in livestock and now began to purchase some outstanding Jersey cattle. By carefully buying a few at a time, he put together a high-quality herd, so good that he entered it in the 1904 World's Fair at Saint Louis with some of the wealthier cattlemen. He brought home a first place award and thirty additional trophies.

The highlight of this World's Fair was the honor signified by a special "Osteopathy Day," an occasion capped with a banquet honoring Osteopathy's founder, Andrew Still. Andrew's former students came from all over the United States and Canada to pay tribute. It was one of the largest banquets held during that World's Fair and significant in that it was the only one at which no liquor was served. While honoring Andrew by their presence, guests showed their great respect for him by seeing that his wishes were carried out and that no liquor was served. This was such a novelty at the time that the Saint Louis newspapers gave the event front-page coverage.

In spite of his honors, Andrew was annoyed with the increased requirements so many state boards were demanding of Osteopathic graduates and disappointed that many former students felt that *materia medica* should be added to ASO's curriculum. As the Old Doctor saw it, teaching the use of drugs in his college violated the basic principles of Osteopathy, and studying something diametrically opposed to his fundamental concept would only dilute student enthusiasm for the principles that made earlier practitioners so successful.

During the second ten years in the operation of the school and hospital, many of the earlier problem areas had been smoothed out and in general now reflected the wishes and philosophy of the founder. The administration, under the able direction of Andrew's eldest son, Charley, had been well tested.

By 1905, many less qualified Osteopathic colleges had closed their doors. Some closed because of inadequate financing, some because they failed to meet Osteopathic college standards. Nearly all those that remained open were upgrading operations to meet standards established by the American Osteopathic Association and state legislatures. ASO had successfully absorbed many of the students from the defunct colleges.

Another type of manipulative therapy was emerging at this time, a method which in some ways derived from the Osteopathic principles established and taught at ASO. In 1896, David D. Palmer visited Kirksville and took some treatments from the Old Doctor. He stayed around for several weeks; and, it's reported, he visited with students and looked over the clinic before he returned to Davenport, Iowa, where he had been practicing as a "magnetic healer." Two years later he opened a school in which he taught his own type of manipulative therapy called chiropractic. For the first several years Palmer's school had only a few students. In 1902, only fifteen students were enrolled. A few years later, only a dozen or so more.

Not until 1906, when Palmer's son B. J. took over the operation of the Davenport school, did the chiropractic movement experience any expansion. B. J. understood the value of advertising and under his aggressive leadership the chiropractic college grew considerably in strength.

By that time, Osteopathy was well established as the pioneer in manipulative medicine and had well-trained graduates practicing under an established state licensing process. Facing this, it took quite a few years for the chiropractic profession to have anything but a minimal impact on the Osteopathic profession.

ASO seemed to be going along smoothly by 1906. It had absorbed many weaker Osteopathic colleges, and had eliminated local competition presented by the Columbia School. Several loyal family members had joined the faculty to remain permanently on the teaching staff and help fill the needs on the staff of the rapidly growing hospital.

It was a great loss when Andrew's nephew, Guy Hulett, who many felt could present the Osteopathic theory better than anyone other than the Old Doctor himself, contracted typhoid fever and died suddenly.

A general feeling of calm and well-being might have continued but for increased competition between the hospital's two general surgeons. At times each exhibited prima donna behavior and expressed negative views of the other's skills and qualifications. Most of all, they were extremely critical and resentful of regulations they felt had been created by individuals who had no surgical training or education.

As vice president of the corporation, Dr. Charley was responsible for the operation of the hospital and had the unenviable task of trying to enforce hospital regulations. Both the battling surgeons had pointed out that they knew a whole lot more about their scope of activity than a group of non-surgically trained board members, and they believed that the surgical regulations were not well thought out and were too restrictive.

Finally one of the surgeons left the hospital staff, leaving only George A. Still, grandson of Jim Still (the brother who had given Andrew such a hard time in the past), as head surgeon. Things quieted down a degree, at least for a while.

By this time, a school to train nurses had been established in the hospital under the supervision of Mary Walters. Now, with many young women in the program, the hospital was well-staffed with nurses and trainees.

In 1908, the cost of a private room with meals varied from fifteen to twenty-five dollars per week. At the same time, a patient staying in the ward would pay only ten dollars a week, with meals.

THE OLD DOCTOR WAS PLEASED with the success of the hospital. He realized the necessity of a facility where patients could receive surgical care and students could observe surgical procedures. He usually considered surgery as a last resort, but was aware that some conditions could only be treated with surgical methods.

Early in his career, Andrew had done a considerable number of minor surgeries in addition to extracting teeth. He also had witnessed many surgeries during his service in the army. Some he considered unnecessary and, for the most part, was disappointed in the results. From those observations, he strengthened his resolve to see that surgery would be used only as a last expedient. This determination made him study even harder to develop ways so a greater number of conditions could be treated without surgical procedures.

With the administrative skills of son Charley, the sound business practices of Warren as business manager, and the financial advice of son Harry, the operation of the school and hospital reached a point where Andrew felt he no longer needed to spend as much time with either and was finally able to devote both time and energy to interests outside his profession.

He decided to stop teaching on a regular basis and only dropped in on classes from time to time. Without having to prepare lectures during his morning walks, he had even more time to use as he chose. And because Mother Still's health, taxed to the breaking point for many years, was slowly deteriorating, Andrew appreciated this new freedom from work and schedules as it gave him more time to spend with her.

Another change, besides losing some of his strength, was taking place in Andrew's life. For many years, most patients arriving in Kirksville came especially to be treated by him.

Now there were excellent practitioners all over the country as well as some with fine reputations in Kirksville. Now patients arrived just to visit with him. They did not expect him to be their doctor.

Although he never considered himself a celebrity, there were many people who came to town merely to meet the discoverer of Osteopathy. There were visitors from foreign countries and some very famous Americans. Among the visitors were two brothers, Robert Love Taylor, twice governor of Tennessee, and his brother, Alfred Alexander Taylor, who would serve as governor of Tennessee in the 1920s. The Taylors thought that since Andrew's middle name was Taylor they might be related, but they were not.

During the next two years, the number of visitors Andrew met with was curtailed because of the progressive deterioration of Mother Still's health. Early in 1907, Andrew became certain that his wife's condition would not improve and, as her health worsened, the full impact of what she meant to him took over all of his thoughts. She had been the helpmate who made so many of his successes possible, as well as the one who carried him through so many adversities.

On his morning walks in previous years, when he was not preparing lectures, he concentrated on the wonders of nature and the universe – stars, animals, plant life, geology. They presented him with so many unanswered questions that he was engrossed in attempting to better understand all the things he saw daily. Recently, the mysteries of life had taken over much of his thinking. In classes he often spoke of Life Force and the mystery of its origin. He had read about meditation and how it allowed one's mind to wander along previously undiscovered pathways. Having no prior experience at meditating, he allowed outside stimuli to disturb his concentration. During the first few weeks of trying to meditate, his notes indicated that he again tried some of the techniques he had attempted ten years earlier when he had delved into spiritualism. At that time he had tried to contact the spirit of an Indian woman named Matah and directed some philosophical questions to her. But as he developed more confidence in his ability to concentrate, he felt he was able to reach out and obtain some answers to his philosophical questions himself.

ANDREW STARTED TO CARRY a small red pocket-sized book that advertised medical products. There was enough space at the bottom of each page for him to jot down a few lines. He probably never planned to share his philosophical observations with anyone, because he rarely corrected his notations. Many notes were apparently written while he was walking since the handwriting is very uneven. In addition, his strange system of abbreviation and his consistently bad spelling made it difficult for a reader to be absolutely certain of his meaning.

Along with his philosophical observations, he wrote lines of poetry, recommendations on diet, and the names of patients with what they had been charged and whether or not they had paid their bills. In some cases, for unknown reasons, he changed the dates from those printed in the book, writing in his own dates. This he did only occasionally.

Most of his poetry was quite clear, however, and so were a few observations which he had taken the trouble to correct. The following is an example of Andrew's poetry:

> Dear little faces, in sunshine and shadow
> Joy causeth your heart e'en to overflow
> You know that cometh a brighter tomorrow,
> Ah, what would it be if it were not so–

Another reads:

> In the noonday of mystery they gathered
> By the side of a deep phantom well.

Wooing the fates that were hidden,
Listing, the future to tell.

Faintly the whisper was wafted
As incense upon the night dew:
Be brave, be courageous, be honest,
To your heart ever be true.

The themes of his philosophical observations were easy to understand since they were repeated several times. He seemed to examine each theme for several weeks. He listed six different themes in his red book: psychic force, realization, purpose, subjugation, concentration, and continuity of thought. Excerpts from his notes on concentration, corrected and fairly legible, follow:

Coming under the heading of distraction, digression, etc., thought as it stands today is the mighty citadel of which the whole universe dwells–

It is the resting place of the mighty whole, but how little it is understood or practiced as it should be–

Thoughts are units of the universe. They go far into making up the creatory force that rules said universe–

The seers of the past were thoughts seekers along the high ways and bye ways of knowledge, ever seeking to imbibe and partake of the grand and revelating utterances of thought that continually surrounded them–

Where are the seers of today that we had in the past? There are none–

This is the fault of distraction in which the world now dwells–

Hence seek ever for the door of concentration. When you have entered therein, let all else go, as the knowledge you seek is contained here and here only.

Another of his themes, continuity of thought, had also been corrected and was fairly legible. It follows:

CONTINUITY OF THOUGHT

Many take up a new line of thought, but lack the continuity of purpose. The slightest excuse draws them from the deviating line, and they are lost.

The first principle contained in continuity is a firm determinance along the will power, safe-guarded by a close concentrated watch over the slightest deviation, or swinging aside of the pendulum of continuous action.

Propose to yourself to arrive at the highest pinnacle of success. If a wondrous amount of wealth was in sight for each and every one of us and we knew that continuity of purpose would lead us eventually to the goal of our ambition, how faithfully and earnestly would we concentrate.

Early progression along this line of thought brings its own reward. It may come in the form of bettering the health condition. It may be in bringing about in the form of greater concentration on business, or in home duties. In a thousand ways such that the instrument find his or herself bettered.

Rehabilitate yourself with the raiment of continuity, carry a fixed purpose for the common good. Continuity of purpose must bring success if concentration accompanies it, for a fixed purpose is the only key to the valley of success where all will be found harmonious through the laws of continuity.

From the dates in his little red book, it appears that Andrew only made notes like these for a period of about six months in 1907, and that he possibly never wrote anything of this nature before or after. His first observation was on the page dated March 11 and the last entry on the page dated September 13. Since there was no attempt on his part to change those dates, they are probably correct.

Miss Per Brown, a librarian who had retired to the Denver area, with the help of three Osteopathic relatives and a psychologist, spent quite a bit of time trying to accurately interpret the writings in the book. Miss Brown wrote of her efforts:

> The haste in which he wrote affected his handwriting. Letters were incomplete, equivocally formed. Words were cramped at the end of the lines, and at the bottom of the pages. A letter, or a word, was in haste mistakenly recorded for one probably intended; "then" for "that," "the" for "they," and "ing" for "ed," for instance.
>
> Realizing this, A. T. sometimes apparently went over some of his writing later. Some corrections show in a sharper pencil and improved handwriting, but he did not catch and change all apparent errors. Aside from the words themselves, the order in which they were recorded presented another difficulty. A. T. used the pages upside down, and a mixture of those. . . .

As careful as Miss Brown and her assistants were, the contents of his observations may not represent Andrew's actual thoughts as they tried to interpret them. The notations may have only been some form of mental exercise that helped him during one of the most stressful periods of his life. Probably the one thing that will always make his meaning unclear was the lack of proper syntax, which could change the total meaning of the statement.

Even before he wrote his last notation in the little red book on September 13, 1907, Andrew had decided that his search for the origin of Life Force was not important enough to take up so much of his time. Maybe, he must have thought, he wasn't supposed to know its origin and even if he did, would it prove to be anything of value?

Recently his wife's health had improved. Her illness stabilized and it appeared that it was not as life threatening as it had been earlier in the year. By the end of August, Andrew again thought about the important and practical things he needed to do. Several times as he sat at his desk, he thought he was ready to begin working again. However, it was not until the middle of September that he actually started work on his projects in earnest.

He had heard that a group of students and a teacher were meeting after class to form a discussion club on spiritualism. He had completely discarded and discredited anything that had to do with contacting spirits. He felt he must do something immediately. He strode angrily into one of the meetings and announced forcefully that "no spirit ever helped me give a treatment or helped me plow a field of corn!"

When he returnd to his room that evening, he told himself to get on with the important things in life as soon as possible. In three years he would be eighty years old and it seemed imperative that he turn all his energy into accomplishing everything of value that he could.

The next morning he sat down at his desk and looked over a pile of material – a collection of unfinished professional articles, sketches of unfinished inventions, unanswered letters, old newspaper articles, and dozens of handwritten notes that had lost their significance.

Andrew was mildly amused when he discovered that he had kept some of his observations dealing with his reaction to human behavior, especially those directed toward pompous egotistical individuals. He had often created a mental picture of a politician becoming so inflated with self-admiration he would actually explode with so much violence it could be heard over a great distance. He remembered he had also assigned preachers and medical doctors to the super-egotist category. He realized he had too much work to do to try to straighten up this mess on his desk at this time. He felt it was imperative to get back to work on his inventions immediately.

As early as 1904, Andrew had constructed a small model of a smokeless furnace. Over the years, he had felt bad about how the residue of coal smoke had so contaminated the country-side and the environment and how, in the wintertime, many of the local buildings had a layer of soot and the snow was turned to a dirty gray.

In 1906 he enlarged his model and incorporated a few minor changes and produced a more efficient model. The principle of his furnace was a specially constructed chamber using a series of reflectors that would force the burning material back into the center of the flame long enough for most of the solid material to be consumed. Then, by adding live steam at exactly the right level into the center of the chamber, nearly all the remaining solids would be burned, leaving the smoke free of carbon particles.

He had demonstrated his smokeless furnace to students and townspeople who suggested that he get it patented as soon as possible. He had one more invention on the drawing board that he could refine while he was going through the patenting process for the furnace. This one was based on the principle of placing a layer of specialized condensing material in the roof of a home. By properly locating this layer, moisture in the air would be condensed and by directing the moisture into a storage tank, extra water – that was also soft water – would be made available.

First, however, he must give most of his attention to getting a patent for his smokeless furnace. In the past, he had seen several of his inventive ideas developed and patented by others. This time, he had not only the time but the desire to develop and patent his smokeless furnace himself.

It took some time before Andrew finally got down to the painful process of hiring a patent attorney. In 1908 he contacted a well-known patent attorney in Chicago, Clarence Taylor, and began preparing sketches, blueprints, and detailed descriptions of the parts. These had to be reviewed many times before a proper presentation for his patent could be made.

By now the Old Doctor was eighty years old. He was reluctant to give so much time to this process as he considered it a matter of minor importance. But details were essential and, finally realizing this, he committed himself to doing whatever was necessary to get his invention – which he considered to be very worthwhile – properly patented. Despite this resolution, he was hardly prepared for how time-consuming the process had become. He had to insure that the sketches were accurately drawn and each part in exact scale. It was necessary to describe the structure as well as the function of each part.

Andrew's attorney pointed out the importance of how his proposal was worded and how essential it was – after a search of patent offices in this country and foreign countries – that his application showed the principle of the operation in such a broad form that his patent would cover a large, general area. Andrew's patience began to wear away with all the correspondence that ensued and the continuous review of his drawings to check their accuracy. He wondered if he would ever get his patent. However, since he could pursue this work at home, he could also spend a great deal of time with his ailing wife. His treatments made her more comfortable and their evening visits made them both feel better.

Andrew had spent several years just thinking through his ideas, a couple of years building and testing his models and making necessary changes. Now with the delays in the patenting process, it was taking even more years to achieve his goal. Finally, on April 26, 1910, all the necessary paperwork was finished and the patent office issued Andrew T. Still a patent for "An Improvement on a Burner."

By the time he received his long-sought certificate that arrived a few days later in the mail, it held little interest for him. His wife had lapsed into a coma and within a month passed away.

MARY ELVIRA HAD BEEN THE BALANCE WHEEL that kept their family functioning as a cohesive unit. With her firm and fair, but gentle method of dealing with family situations before they became serious problems, she had often been sought out for her advice. Her patience and wisdom had guided many of Andrew's projects to completion.

As the Still children were gathered for the funeral, they agreed that their mother had been one of the main reasons that Osteopathy had finally been developed and that a great deal of their father's success had resulted from the contributions of Mother Still. They agreed to share the family responsibilities in the months ahead. Blanche felt she could look after her father. Charley, who lived next door, said he would help her. Harry, who was about to return to live in Kirksville, would also be available to help. Herman stayed in Kirksville for several months and since he was mechanically inclined – having constructed some complicated gadgets and machinery – he was to assist Andrew in promoting his invention.

Following his wife's death, Andrew did little to promote the furnace. He turned it over to a large company, but when they increased it to a commercial size, it didn't perform like the original model that had performed perfectly in its many tests.

Herman and Andrew heard about the failures and discussed some of the reasons it might have failed. Andrew doubted that the company had placed the reflectors at exactly the right angles and might also have failed to place the jets for the live steam at the right level. They both agreed that the principle was correct and that a good mechanical engineer should be able to make these corrections.

After a trip to the company, Herman reported that the people there didn't seem very interested in following his and Andrew's suggestions by making any changes. Instead, they scrapped the idea of manufacturing the furnace.

As disappointed as the Old Doctor was with this failure after all the time and hard work he had invested in the furnace design, he no longer had the energy to make the necessary corrections to successfully market his invention himself.

Herman had no marketing experience and wanted to return to his practice in Texas. Regretfully, Andrew put his invention away, stating that sometime in the future he would find the right company to fully develop the furnace he considered a truly outstanding and beneficial discovery.

At the same time he had been tinkering with his smokeless furnace, he was also thinking about a three-week visit he had made to the state mental hospital in Nevada, Missouri. While observing the patients there, he had manipulated quite a few and apparently with some success.

With his institution in Kirksville doing so well, he came to the conclusion that it was about time to consider building or setting up some type of sanatorium where mental patients could receive proper manipulative therapy. For a while, at least, he decided to concentrate on developing such an institution and put all thoughts of his inventions aside.

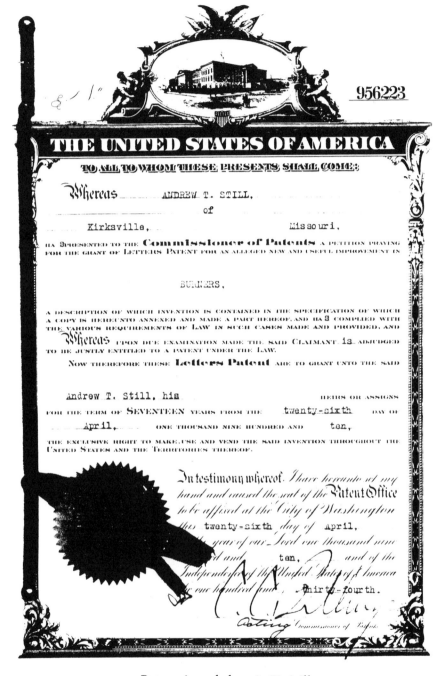

Patent Awarded to A. T. Still

Chapter Sixteen

VEN BEFORE HIS MOTHER'S DEATH, Dr. Charley realized that his responsibilities would be increasing for many years. He was already serving as the administrative head of both the school and the hospital and, except for an official title, was also acting president of the corporation owning both facilities.

During the last days of his mother's illness, many returning graduates had come to his house next door after visiting with the Old Doctor. Most considered themselves members of the family and expected to be fed and, in some cases, to be housed as well. The antiquated home where he and his family were living was clearly inadequate to properly entertain the great number of visitors to the college. He knew that Blanche would continue to care for their father and see that his declining strength was not overextended, but she was in no position to do much entertaining.

So Charley and his wife, Anna, decided early in 1909 to build a new home, one large enough and modern enough to meet the growing demands of their social obligations. The difficulty was finding enough money. Although Dr. Charley's income from operating the school and from his obstetrical practice was sufficient for them to live well, it was hardly enough to build a new house.

The only solution was to sell the Jersey herd he had assembled over the previous eight years. He had already considered reducing the herd's size because he was having trouble hiring farm help. Now, to raise sufficient capital for the dream house, he would have to sell the entire herd, not just a few head. Some of his animals had won grand championships and first and second place awards in state and national competitions, but until he put them on the market he wouldn't know their actual value.

He contacted several of the wealthiest members of the American Jersey Cattle Association. Two in particular already had fine herds and were anxious to acquire some of Charley's outstanding cattle. They told him they would purchase most of his stock and pay a good price if he would do something for them.

The buyers recognized Dr. Charley's widespread reputation as a good breeder of Jersey cattle. Knowing that Charley and his family would like to go to Europe to see the Passion Play, they offered not only to buy his cattle but help pay for much of a European trip if Charley would visit the Isle of Jersey and bring back fifty good animals for them.

Assured that the sale of the Jersey herd would bring in enough money to build their new home, Anna and Charley spent many hours planning what they would like to have in it. Anna also worked with the architect in drawing up the plans. The goal was to have a home that would serve the family and be a place ASO alumni could use, a home they could be proud of as the residence of the acting chief administrator.

Plans were put on hold because Mother Still's health was precarious and she was not expected to live through the winter. After she passed away that spring of 1910, and following several strategy meetings between Andrew and his children, Anna and Charley finalized the details of their trip to Europe and to see the Passion Play.

IN JULY 1910, DR. CHARLEY AND ANNA, daughters Gladys and Elizabeth, and son Charley, Jr., traveled by train to New

York. There they boarded the luxurious Cunard liner *Mauritania,* sister ship of the ill-fated *Lusitania,* and traveled on to England.

The family toured France, Holland, and Switzerland, then attended the Passion Play in Oberammergau, Germany. They returned to London and rented a flat for three months. Dr. Charley spent much of his time on the Isle of Jersey, negotiating the best price on choice Jersey cattle.

Four months later, ending their European stay, the Still family boarded a not-so-glamorous cattle boat, and along with fifty-five head of Jersey cattle, they headed for New York. On arriving in the United States, the family was met by representatives of C. I. Hood of Lowell, Massassachusetts, and the Rockefellers. The party congratulated Dr. Charley on a job well done and took possession of the animals, keeping some for their own herds and selling the remainder to other cattlemen.

After his return to Kirksville, Dr. Charley was criticized for taking so much time away from his job. Some people were apparently jealous of anyone who could travel to Europe at this time. However, he felt the school and hospital had been, and were, in good hands. Brother Harry was in the process of moving back to Kirksville and George Laughlin and his wife Blanche had seen that the family interests were well represented. Even the Old Doctor was healthy enough to help if there had been any important decisions to be made. He felt he had been tied down to the operation of the school since its inception and was justified in taking a long vacation.

Dr. Charley soon learned the sale of his cattle herd was not sufficient to cover the cost of building the new house, which was exceeding original estimates. He found it necessary to sell some of his interest in the farm on the east end of town where he had kept his herd to brother-in-law George Laughlin. Because he loved his livestock, he kept four Jersey cows which he claimed were to supply his family and guests with fresh milk and cream.

DURING DR. CHARLEY'S ABSENCE, Andrew had busied himself with planning an institution to treat mental patients who, he felt certain, would improve with properly applied manipulative therapy in a pleasant environment.

Finally, in 1913 the exceptionally well-constructed Blees Military Academy in Macon, Missouri became available. Located on nearly four hundred acres of rolling countryside with two lakes, a main building, and an annex, it would – with a few modifications – house two hundred patients. There was also a fine home on the property about half a mile from the main building. It would make an ideal home for the superintendent.

This was exactly the type of setup Andrew had envisioned. He sincerely believed that mental patients could improve if they ate appetizing, nutritious food, were given physical and recreational activities, heard good music, had good books to read, were kept well groomed and – not least important – were surrounded by a friendly staff who further encouraged them.

Dr. Hildreth was named as president and superintendent, Dr. Charley as vice president, and Dr. Harry as secretary and treasurer. The Still-Hildreth Sanitarium opened during the first week in March 1914. The Old Doctor had seen another of his goals attained and could hardly wait to see the results that the new institution would achieve.

In his dedication address, Andrew gazed at the beauty of this new institution and spoke glowingly of the potential for changing the treatment of mental patients. He predicted that this institution would lead the way to better and more humane care of patients with mental problems.

From its inception, Still-Hildreth Sanitarium was a successful operation. This was at a time when most mental hospitals and sanatoriums were simply locking their patients away. Patients were rarely seen by a doctor and had little or no physical or recreational opportunities. This new Osteopathic sanatorium provided its patients with manipulation therapy three times a week and encouraged patients to participate in recreational activities. During the summer, many took regular walks, pitched horseshoes, played tennis, or tossed a baseball around. In the winter, the billiard room and music room were popular spots. Quite a few played dominoes and often several card games were in progress. The barbershop and beauty shop were also popular.

It was not long before Still-Hildreth was receiving patients from nearly every state. Although the sanatorium was only a couple of miles from the Wabash station in Macon, there were soon so many travelers coming to Still-Hildreth that the railroad began making regular passenger stops at a small building just outside the main gate. On the Wabash Railroad map this stop was listed as "Hildreth."

The year of 1914 had been a good one for the Osteopathic profession in northern Missouri and for the Still family in particular. The sanatorium opened in Macon, and the hospital in Kirksville gained more space with the addition of a fourth floor. The hospital building was also totally renovated on the inside and a new tile roof added much to its exterior appearance.

The hospital business was growing rapidly. Dr. George Still had proved to be an outstanding general surgeon, and Dr. George Laughlin was developing his reputation as an innovative orthopedic surgeon. There were times, however, when the Old Doctor questioned the fact that so much surgery was being performed in this Osteopathic hospital. Dr. Charley was acting as his spokesman and watchdog, but there were times when Dr. George still felt he was being criticized unjustly for doing too much surgery.

Being both a talented and personable young man, George often felt too restrained in his work by the regulations the board imposed. He stated that the quality of his work might be affected if he were not allowed more leeway. He had a medical degree and he had earlier contemplated making the old Columbia School, which he had purchased, into a medical school. However, this created such a furor among those in the Osteopathic profession that he dropped the idea.

The year 1914 had also proven successful for the ASO baseball team, undefeated for the first time against strong opposition. Charley, Jr., was the mascot. The team featured a former New York Giants pitcher, Cecil Ferguson, as the number one man of a strong pitching staff.

During the same year, another major project came to fruition. During the National Osteopathic Convention in Kirksville in 1913, a decision had been made to erect a statue of the Old Doctor, which would hopefully be completed during his lifetime. Plans for the statue had been developing for several years, and much of the momentum to ensure that it be completed as soon as possible had come from the Sojourner's Club. The club was quickly supported in this effort by the Still family, as well as by many members of the Osteopathic profession. George Julian Zolnay, a noted artist and sculptor, was commissioned for the project, but fund-raising had stalled. For a period of time even the heroic efforts of the Sojourner's members to get the statue finished faced failure.

Finally, Dr. George Still, who had great respect for his Great Uncle Andrew in spite of their differing views on the value of surgery, took it upon himself to get the profession behind the project so that Andrew, the founder of Osteopathy, could be present at the dedication and unveiling of the statue honoring him. There was much concern that if they didn't concentrate their efforts on raising the money necessary to complete the statue soon enough, the Old Doctor might not be present for such a dedication. This worry gave the money raisers motivation to really bear down on their effort.

Although Dr. Charley's new home had been completed late in 1912, it took over a year to get the twenty-four-room home properly furnished. It was in the spring of 1914 before Anna Still had everything in order so she could entertain visiting alumni and local residents. She was especially proud of the large dining room with a table that could seat twenty-four people. There were many other special features: a parlor for her daughters on the first floor, a ballroom on the third floor large enough for fifty or more couples, a dumbwaiter that connected all three floors, an interfloor intercom system that included the basement where a central vacuum system with a large motor was housed and most rooms were equipped with round vents in the baseboards to which vacuum hoses could be connected.

Anna's dream house had become a reality. She had planned it well. Her home was beautiful, outside and in, and she could now entertain all guests. Many visitors were eager to view all the innovations in the new house.

A final highlight of 1914 for Dr. Charley was being elected mayor of Kirksville. This civic duty was in addition to his duties at the college. Anna and Charley felt they had planned well for the responsibilities they would face in the future.

However, all of the year's successes were clouded in the late fall when Andrew suffered a slight stroke. Although he soon made a satisfactory recovery, it was easy to see that he had lost quite a bit of his already reduced vitality. Nonetheless, by the beginning of 1915, Andrew was once again seeing and visiting with the many people who came to Kirksville expressly to see him.

Among his famous guests were Helen Keller, who along with her companion, spent a couple of days visiting the school and witnessing the growth of the institution after having a long and serious discussion with Andrew.

Andrew loved to have his visitors meet with him on the front porch of his home. As soon as the winter weather abated, it was a common sight to see Andrew and his guests having what he often referred to as a powwow in plain view of passersby. Some of these discussions were obviously very serious.

Buffalo Bill's Wild West Show came to Kirksville, which gave William Cody an opportunity to have a long visit with the Old Doctor on his front porch and the chance to have brunch with Dr. Charley and his family. This was a real thrill for the Still children, especially young Charley, Jr., who was invited to attend the performance as Buffalo Bill's special guest.

William Cody's father, Isaac, had served in the early Kansas legislature as speaker of the house. He was such a strong abolitionist that he and the Still family had much in common. However, Cody's father was less fortunate than Abram Still, and he was fatally stabbed while making an antislavery speech.

Cody had tried during an earlier visit in 1911 to visit the Old Doctor, but the two had been unable to make connections. This time, they spent more than an hour together and had a chance to discuss much of the turbulent history of Kansas.

Even though the Old Doctor continued to see as many visitors as his daughter would allow, there was little doubt that his health was deteriorating. This prompted Dr. George Still to make a quick trip to Washington, D.C. to make an additional payment on the statue, to inspect its progress, and to urge George Zolnay to speed up his timetable for completion.

Upon his return, George devoted himself to raising the money for the final payment. He suggested that each student contribute at least one dollar to the effort and he contacted many of the local businessmen for an additional contribution. He repeated his strong belief in *ante mortem* tributes and stressed to the students how wonderful it would be for the Old Doctor to hear that every single student had contributed to the fund. Once the fund-raising effort gained momentum, Dr. George was able to return to his surgical practice.

Dr. George Still had gained a reputation in northern Missouri as an outstanding and progressive surgeon. On December 6, 1915, he quite suddenly achieved national fame. An ASO student was depressed and tried to end his life by shooting himself in the heart. Dr. George opened the man's chest and removed the bullet that had passed through the heart. After removing the accumulated blood from the pericardial sack, he massaged the heart slowly and carefully. With the relieved pressure and the gentle massage, the heart started beating normally. Dr. George then carefully sutured the wound and closed the chest. The patient made an uneventful recovery.

All of this was done without any mechanical aid or transfusion and without a team of specially trained surgeons and nurses to give Dr. George assistance. Not only did the local and state newspapers cover the event, but many national papers also carried the story of this daring and successful surgical achievement.

ALTHOUGH HE WAS RIDING A CREST OF POPULARITY, Dr. George at times felt frustrated. He felt the hospital and school would progress more rapidly if they were run by someone with a more progressive attitude. When he had purchased the Columbia School with the thought of developing a progressive Osteopathic school, he was disappointed that so many ASO alumni had reacted so negatively. He was also aware that Dr. Charley was in a position to become the president of the organization that operated the school and hospital after the passing of the Old Doctor. Andrew had also publicly stated that he would like his school to remain in the hands of his immediate family. That meant that at least for the foreseeable future Dr. Charley would head the operation.

Many of Dr. George Still's friends and admirers, after hearing him express his frustration, suggested that if he could acquire additional stock in the company, he could reach his goal of being president. In that way, he could establish a more progressive school and hospital operation. They also pointed out that Dr. Charley would occasionally sell some of his own stock to meet his changing financial requirements.

Dr. Charley had heard that some of Dr. George's friends were eager for him to become president of the company. Although he had great respect for his cousin's surgical ability, he felt that because of lack of administrative experience, George would hardly be qualified to operate the college. Charley also felt that he, on the other hand, had enough experience dealing with personnel that, once he didn't have to follow his father's dictates to the letter, he would be able to work out things so the two of them could work well together.

Charley also knew that some of Dr. George's friends had bought some stock in the company, so he decided that if and when he had to put some of his own stock up for sale, it would only go to the immediate family or to friends he could trust totally. Dr. Charley had spent a great deal of his life working to become the president of ASO. He certainly did not plan on doing anything to jeopardize his chance to reach that goal.

Sometimes Charley was not too happy with the comments of some of Dr. George's cronies, particularly when they stated he was not aggressive enough to supervise the progressive changes that ASO must make in the future. He had actually been thinking that, at some time in the future, tuition fees would not meet the total cost of an improved educational program. Sooner or later, he felt, in order to meet the expanding needs for better teachers and more modern facilities, the alumni would have to help, not only in planning, but also in providing some financial support.

Dr. Charley had realized that in the past there might have been some justification for claiming that he had too many outside interests. It had been for this reason that he sold his interest in the Star Coal Mine to some local businessmen. Furthermore, his Jersey herd had been reduced to just enough animals to supply his family and the hospital with milk.

He felt that now he would have more time to concentrate on the college and planning for its future. He had spent nearly twenty-five years supervising and watching the school grow from seventeen students to nearly a thousand. He was extremely proud that he could call so many graduates by their first names.

With the exception of Dr. Hildreth, he had attended more state Osteopathic conventions and helped more state organizations when they requested it than anyone else. He knew that the school he envisioned would certainly need the help of the alumni he had grown close to over the years in order to help guarantee the continued quality expansion of ASO.

Dr. Charley wondered if some of Dr. George's ardent admirers really thought this young surgeon with no administrative experience could step in and properly operate a college that had survived so many crises under his own guidance. George had been only ten years old when the first class came to Kirksville. Dr. Charley put the thought out of his mind. He doubted that anyone, other than the young doctor's closest friends, would feel George could take on such a demanding job.

Once again, Dr. Charley ran for mayor and received a strong vote of confidence. With his political position and his house ready to meet any social requirement, he and Anna felt they were now in a position to make their home a place to entertain students, faculty, alumni, and visiting dignitaries.

Since his mother, Mary Elvira, had attended college in Poughkeepsie, New York, Charley hoped one of his daughters might someday attend Vassar. He was very happy when his eldest daughter, Gladys, was accepted at that prestigious institution.

The National Convention of the American Osteopathic Association was held in the summer of 1916 at Kansas City. Since it was not too far from Kirksville, the meeting gave a large number of Osteopaths another chance to visit the college and pay their respects to their founder. The Old Doctor was pleased that so many of his "children," as he called his former students, would make the extra effort to come to Kirksville before, during, or following the convention.

AS THE SUMMER OF 1916 CAME TO A CLOSE, war clouds in Europe were becoming more ominous by the day. Sometimes, on the warm evenings of late summer and early fall as the Still family sat on the front porch of their new home, members of the college Glee Club would gather in front of the nurse's cottage to serenade nurses and trainees. Much of the music had the sentimental, bittersweet lyrics that were so characteristic of the World War I era. The fine male voices, rendering many of the sentimental songs, were often joined by several banjo players.

Almost the only sounds besides the music were the laughter of musicians and young ladies being serenaded, the occasional noise of a lone automobile, or the rare squeal of tires as Dr. George, in his usual hurry to surgery, came down Osteopathy Avenue too rapidly and tried to negotiate the turn into the hospital parking lot. Everything seemed so perfect that it was hard to believe the United States would in a short time be plunged into a foreign war.

Chapter Seventeen

ANUARY AND FEBRUARY OF 1917 seemed extremely cold to Andrew Still. It was hard to keep the house warm enough for him to leave the comfort of his bed. In an effort to warm him, Blanche kept the house so hot that her husband and daughter could barely stand staying indoors. Nonetheless, Andrew felt chilled during the brief periods he stayed out of bed. He knew his statue was completed and would soon be shipped to Kirksville. He also knew a date had been set for the unveiling ceremonies. But he seemed more interested in wishing the cold weather would go away so that his joints would move without so much pain.

March wasn't much warmer. If Andrew didn't improve, the organizers of the unveiling ceremonies, in addition to several hundred alumni, friends, and distinguished guests, might not see the Old Doctor attend this special event that was to honor him for his lifetime of service and accomplishments.

It was not until mid-April that the Old Doctor perked up enough to show some interest in the activities. One sunny afternoon, sitting on his front porch bundled up against the weather, he watched workmen set up the base for the statue and he soon became involved in some of the excitement that had gripped the Still family for weeks. He called his daughter aside and joked about being one of the very few men who would see a statue dedicated to himself. He also told her he doubted if his accomplishments justified anything of this magnitude.

The one thing he felt extremely proud of was that he had created a profession that truly benefited women and that, among the six thousand graduates of his school, there were now a great number of successful women practitioners. He was sorry that no blacks had yet chosen to enter his profession, especially since he had welcomed them from the beginning.

Andrew was also proud that there were now D.O.'s practicing in all forty-eight states, as well as in several foreign countries. It had recently been reported that the Littlejohn brothers were starting an Osteopathic college in London. With ASO graduates acting as medical missionaries in India and Africa and recent practitioners locating in Australia, Andrew now saw his dream come true and, in less than twenty-five years, his profession had circled the globe.

Dr. George Still, who had been so instrumental in raising funds so the sculpture could be completed and in supervising the timely completion of the work, was in charge of the dedication program. The statue was placed on the hospital lawn on the northeast corner of Osteopathy Avenue and Jefferson Street. Andrew had been to the site in a wheelchair a couple of times and as May 23 approached he said he was sure that he could sit through the whole ceremony in a chair without too much trouble.

As the large crowd gathered, Andrew walked, with some help, from his house to a chair on Dr. Charley's front lawn. From there he had a clear view of the proceedings. His daughter, Blanche Laughlin, stood by his side and his young granddaughter, three-year-old Mary Jane Laughlin, held his hand during part of the ceremonies. His ten-year-old grandson, Charley, Jr., had the privilege of pulling the cord that unveiled the statue.

The sculptor, Zolnay, had portrayed Andrew in the outfit that he wore so often: boots with his pants tucked in, slouch hat, and a long staff in his hand. The inscription on the base was one of Andrew's quotations: "The God I worship demonstrates all His work."

Many of the alumni who attended the ceremony were saddened to see their former teacher, whom they remembered as a man of such vitality, in a feeble state of health. Nonetheless, they were pleased that he had been able to see his statue unveiled in his lifetime, a rare event.

In deference to the Old Doctor's frailty, the program was very brief. Dr. John R. Kirk, president of the Normal School, introduced the Honorable John Swanger, the legislator who had helped with the passage of the Osteopathic bill in Missouri.

The Old Doctor seemed to enjoy the proceedings. At the end of the ceremony, he stood up and waved to the crowd as he left the chair he had been sitting in and then returned to his home in a wheelchair.

The family and all in attendance congratulated Dr. George for putting on such an excellent program, as well as for his fund-raising efforts. The Sojourners Club was also thanked for its effort.

Many among the crowd were saddened as they left, since they realized this would probably be the last time Dr. Andrew Taylor Still, the Old Doctor, would appear in public.

ONE OF DR. CHARLEY'S LONG-TERM AMBITIONS had been to own the largest and most powerful automobile in Kirksville. So, in late 1916, he had ordered a Pierce Arrow 66 Series touring car, which at that time was the largest automobile made in America. A few years later, President Taft visited Kirksville and claimed that the Pierce Arrow Dr. Charley owned was the only car in which he felt he could spread out and be comfortable.

Dr. Charley had hoped the new car would be delivered early enough for the unveiling of his father's statue, but it was nearly midsummer of 1917 before it arrived in Kirksville Automobiles were still such a novelty then that the family eagerly anticipated the car. When it arrived, all the family members were excited and impressed by the power and size of the car when they took it for its first ride. The car was actually so long that on some of the downtown streets it was necessary to back up at least once to negotiate a sharp corner.

In the summer of 1917, Dr. Charley and his family prepared for their first long trip in the Piece Arrow to attend the American Osteopathic Association's National Convention in Columbus, Ohio. Even though he had seen many associates and old friends at the statue unveiling, he was looking forward to seeing his friends in the profession once again and discussing the growth and future of Osteopathy with them.

As the family loaded into the car and headed east for the convention, Dr. Charley realized he had been so immersed in his work and concerns for his father's health for so long that he hadn't noticed his daughter's listlessness. Gladys hadn't been her usual buoyant self since her return from Vassar in early June. As they drove through eastern Illinois, they ran into rainstorms. At mud holes, members of the family had to get out and do some pushing. On their second night of travel, after a difficult day, they were cleaning up in a small town hotel when Gladys complained that she wasn't feeling very well. As she started for her room, she had a massive hemorrhage that seemed to originate from her lungs.

Dr. Charley and his wife realized they had a seriously ill daughter. Attending the convention, that had seemed so important, required more courage than they had thought would be possible, but they would keep their chins up when they greeted old friends.

The trip back to Missouri gave them time to realize that they now had another worry besides the Old Doctor's frail health that had occupied them for so many months. Their talented and beautiful daughter had contracted tuberculosis and was in a serious condition.

THE WAR HAD NOT BEEN IN PROGRESS VERY LONG before college administrators began to see that it was going to have a strong impact on the school. Many of the patriotic graduates of recent classes had applied to join the armed forces and sought commissions in the Medical Corps. They were terribly disappointed when this request was denied. Quite a few did go ahead and enlist in the army, navy, and marine corps to serve in whatever capacity was assigned them.

What really disturbed senior students and recent graduates was that nurses who graduated from the Osteopathic Nursing School were being accepted and were serving in the military as officers, in spite of the fact that they had much less training and education than ASO graduates. As a result, during the fall semester of 1917, there was a great decline in the number of students enrolling in the Kirksville institution.

Throughout that autumn, Dr. Charley watched helplessly as Gladys' health declined. Nothing he did seemed to help. After discussing the situation with his wife, they decided that Gladys should spend some time in a warmer, drier climate. Anna and Gladys left for San Antonio shortly after Thanksgiving, intending to spend the winter there. Meanwhile, Andrew's health continued to decline.

Dr. Charley was spending more time planning changes that would be necessary to bring the school back to its full operational capacity. He found the time through a variety of factors. The sanatorium in Macon was doing so well it required very little attention from him, new government regulations had closed the Star Mine on his property, he no longer had show animals to tend, and his job as mayor kept him in Kirksville.

Being in charge of the decision making since the inception of the school had given him a good perspective on the changes nearly all colleges would necessarily face in the future. He was fairly sure that the days of a stock company operating a college for profit would not continue for long. Spiraling costs would certainly eat up any profits. This was one reason he spent so much time staying in contact with the alumni. He had been careful to listen to their complaints and suggestions and act on them when they were justified.

He was not too pleased when some of Dr. George's cronies suggested that, since he was not treating patients or doing surgery and had reduced his obstetrical practice, he was not earning his salary. He wondered how anyone could think that the administration of a college was only a part-time job. He felt he had a full-time job, and that he must do all the planning necessary, and everything else he could, to see that the institution his father had founded remained the best Osteopathic college. Actually, when he was delivering more babies, he had earned quite a bit more money than he was making in this "part-time" job.

He dismissed the rumor that the group surrounding Dr. George had convinced George to go after the presidency of the college after the Old Doctor's death. The only person who controlled enough stock to make this a possibility was the widow of Warren Hamilton.

Dr. Charley felt that Mrs. Hamilton was so well informed about how her husband and he had successfully battled through so many crises and how the two had strained together to keep faculty, students, and alumni happy, that there was no possibility she would risk her large investment on a man with no administrative experience, a man whose time was already stretched to the limit performing surgeries.

Although Andrew's health improved for two or three months during the summer of 1917, as soon as cool weather arrived he began losing ground rapidly. He had suffered a few light strokes, but had been able to recover from them until a major stroke in early December that caused his death on December 12.

Even though the immediate family knew Andrew's death was imminent, they were still shocked when it finally arrived. Blanche Laughlin had been so close to her father, and had practically worshiped him, that it was particularly hard on her. Dr. Harry and Dr. Charley, who had tried to follow their father's wishes, joined their sister in her grief for the passing of the gentle, kind man who was known as "Daddy," or "Pap," to thousands of former students, patients, and friends.

At this time, Dr. Charley's wife, Anna, was in San Antonio with their daughter Gladys, and they decided the two should not risk returning to Kirksville and the cold weather, so the women did not make the trip to attend the funeral.

Because so many had attended the unveiling of the statue earlier that year and there was a war going on which made travel difficult, most of those at the funeral were from the local area. Other colleges and the American Osteopathic Association were also well represented.

Thousands of letters from all over the world showed clearly that this kind, dedicated man had left a legacy of accomplishment that truly encircled the globe. Dr. Charley and his sister Blanche assumed the arduous task of answering the flood of personal condolences.

EARLY IN 1918, THE INFLUENZA EPIDEMIC sweeping Europe found its way to the United States and finally to the Midwest. Many of the D.O.'s, who had been treating respiratory infections successfully with manipulation, used the same procedure to treat the pneumonia that so often was a complication of this strain of Spanish flu.

The flu patients, who received manipulation and were under the care of an Osteopathic physician, had such a low mortality rate compared to those under medical care that the American Osteopathic Association decided to document the results from more than 2,400 reporting D.O.'s. The results indicated that "pure" Osteopathy lowered the mortality rate dramatically.

There was little doubt that there would have been fewer flu deaths if more Americans had had the advantage of Osteopathic care. Instead, this epidemic killed more than half a million residents of the United States, in addition to another fifty thousand American troops in Europe.

Many D.O.'s who treated large numbers of flu patients successfully also treated their own families who had been exposed to the flu as a preventive measure. They reported their families had no complications of the disease. A high percentage showed they didn't have even slight cases of flu. This success was reinforced by the fact that so many untreated friends contracted the disease and, in many cases, hadn't shown the immunity evidenced by the Osteopathic families.

The result of these Osteopathic successes introduced many more families to Osteopathy, a badly needed boost to the profession at that time.

WITH A BOARD MEETING SCHEDULED for mid-January of 1918, Dr. Charley took time out from reading and replying to all the letters of sympathy to work on the presentation he planned to make before the board. He had many ideas on what he considered necessary changes the board should hear.

He worked long and hard on his lengthy report. He had discounted rumors that Dr. George was positioning himself to take over the reins of the school. Dr. Charley felt that George was smart enough to realize his successes in surgery hardly qualified him to be administrator of the college, especially during the period of crisis it was currently experiencing. He felt secure, also, that Mrs. Hamilton, who held the pivotal shares of stock, had the reputation of being a good business-woman. He doubted she would place her sizable financial investment in the hands of someone who had no actual experience in guiding a college.

As he called the board meeting to order, he was completely stunned when a motion was made that he not be considered for the presidency. Then Mrs. Hamilton cast her vote representing her large block of stock to make this vote binding. If Dr. Charley had looked around the room, he would have seen that several other board members were also in shock.

He knew other board members were aware that he had been working on a report on his methods and recommendations to improve the operation of the school and hospital. They, too, were stunned since they had not been informed about a potential leadership change. Unfortunately, they didn't represent enough voting shares to make any difference.

There was no chance for him to discuss his plans for the future of the college. When he left the meeting, he was hardly aware of the friends who gathered around him to suggest that, after the board thought it over, it might want to change its vote and offer him the presidency.

The full realization of what had happened soon took over his thoughts. It obviously had been a power play in which Mrs. Hamilton had been convinced the college would progress more under new leadership. Never in his wildest dreams had Charley considered the possibility that Mrs. Hamilton would not support him.

For a few days following the meeting, Dr. Charley sat at the window of his second-story bedroom, looking down on the hospital and the campus of the college he now felt sure he would never serve as president. He finally turned his thoughts back to the present. There were three things to be done.

Perhaps the most difficult was to call his wife in San Antonio to tell her of the board's action and how it would totally change their lives. Also, he had to protect his financial interests, and he must strive to protect the future of the college which his father founded and he himself had shepherded for so many years. He felt he should file a suit to protect these interests because he was afraid that, if the school didn't have proper management, his stock would become worthless. He also felt his salary as vice president should continue to be paid since he had not been notified he had been terminated.

Fortunately, these issues were settled out of court. He now had no financial interest in the school and could spend time reducing the divisiveness caused by his dismissal as administrator. Before he could minimize the bitterness that he, his friends, and his family felt, he decided he must analyze why it had happened.

He had been aware that Dr. George had been acquiring additional stock, but he had been sure that he and his sister, along with Mrs. Hamilton, would always have control of the majority of voting shares since he would be certain never to sell enough of his stock to allow others to gain a majority.

He expected that, sometime in the future, George Still, as a minority stockholder, would come to him and they could work on ways to give him a voice in the operation of the institution.

In retrospect, his only mistake had been to place his trust in Mrs. Hamilton. He had been in the Hamilton home often. He had helped her husband during his final illness, even taking him to Florida in an effort to improve his health. Her support now of the opposition seemed like a bad dream. It was totally unbelievable.

It would later be claimed that one reason for firing him was that he was too busy with outside interests, but at the time the board met, there were no grounds for that accusation. If there was anything to fault him for it was that he had worked so closely with his previous business managers – first Henry Patterson, then Warren Hamilton. He had always worked with the business manager as a team on a day-to-day basis. Working together so closely, he had been able to anticipate problems that might develop and resolve them before they became too difficult.

When the new business manager took over after Warren Hamilton's death in 1911, there was quite a backlog of paperwork left from Warren's long illness. It was early in 1912 before Gene Brott took over as secretary and treasurer of the corporation. It took so long to get everything in order that Brott never took on the additional and more comprehensive role of his predecessors. This left a gap in the school's operation. This is what Dr. Charley had planned to discuss with the board during the January meeting. He had felt he needed an assistant to help him with the continuous supervision of college operations.

Because of his daughter's illness and his father's frailty, Charley had seen only a few board members regularly. He had planned opening additional dialogue with all of them once he had assumed his new position and he wasn't surprised when the board offered the presidency to George Laughlin. He knew it was a token gesture.

Knowing how bitter his sister was about his firing, Charley felt it was a certainty that her husband would refuse the job. Dr. George Still was not sure that he was ready to take on the job either, with all its added responsibilities. So for several months, the college struggled along without a president.

Besides a falling enrollment, there were other problems. Several faculty members, who felt a deep loyalty to Dr. Charley, quit, or announced their intention to do so. The alumni reaction was fairly predictable. Many of the early graduates, who knew Dr. Charley personally, were unhappy over the firing, and worried about the future of their school. More recent graduates, who knew Dr. George, felt he had the potential leadership qualities and that he might be able to develop a more progressive institution. Unfortunately, there was much bitterness within the profession.

In Kirksville, Dr. Charley had been a popular mayor and had been in charge of the school for so long that many local people supported his position. But there was an equal number who gave their complete support to Dr. George and his popular wife, Ardella.

DR. CHARLEY WANTED TO STAY AS FAR AWAY from the bitterness as possible. He now only felt saddened by what had happened, so decided to stay in his home and go through all of the letters that had arrived, not only after his father's death, but also the hundreds he had received after the January board meeting. He was pleased that so many of the former students had taken the time to write to tell him that they, too, were saddened that he had not been elected to the presidency of their college. Many of the letters recounted the early struggles of the school and the profession. Nearly all had spoken of the kindness, patience, and inspirational influence of the Old Doctor.

One letter that had arrived after his father's death reminded him of the growth of his profession, and the many people who had benefited from Osteopathy. During the time that he was staying away from all of the local controversy, he decided to reread this one letter that had so impressed him. This particular letter not only included all of the kind things that had been said by so many, but also pointed out so well how far the profession had come in such a few years.

The woman writing stated that in 1892, as a girl of seventeen, she had been brought to Kirksville to see the Old Doctor. She was not only suffering from persistent headaches, but had not been able to walk for two years following a fall.

After her parents helped her out of the buggy, Dr. Still came out of the house and carried her, with the help of her mother, into his office, which was then a small room in his home containing only a pine board table covered by a blanket, a few chairs, and a bag of bones. Andrew had lifted the frail girl onto the table, all the while studying her facial expression.

He asked the girl's mother a few questions and then, quite suddenly, said, "She is worth saving. You could well afford to give up your farm to have her cured."

The mother told Andrew they had no farm. He then asked her to go out and talk to her husband for a moment. While she was away, Andrew turned to the girl and said, "It makes no difference. I will treat you anyway."

When the mother returned, he began running his fingers up and down the girl's spine, reflecting aloud, "If you were setting out onions, you would say that this one is out of the row."

He gave the girl a gentle treatment and said, "This is all for today. I want to see you in a month," adding that he would take them around to the Miller house where they could have dinner.

"I have only one wife," he remarked, laughing, "and if I kill her feeding all of the people who come to see me, I cannot get another."

The Old Doctor and the father supported the young girl between them. When they reached the steps of the Miller house, Andrew picked her up as if she were a child and set her down at the table. He gave her an autographed photograph of himself and said good-bye.

The next morning the girl awoke with a cry of joy, "My head does not ache!" It was the first time in two years.

In a month, she returned to Kirksville and remained in Andrew's home for the following six months. He had a small bed in the corner of the living room, which he gave up to her because she could not climb the stairs.

The girl, now a woman, wrote:

> It was there that I became acquainted with his wonderful family. Mother Still was truly a mother in every sense of the word. It was a great privilege to know the Old Doctor, both as a friend and a benefactor. He had a wonderful personality, a very forgiving spirit, was generous to a fault.
>
> He treated me frequently, rolling me from the bed across his knees by putting his hands under my frail body. He continued to treat me regularly, even though I did not improve for the first three months.
>
> His brother, Dr. Ed Still, told him sever times, "Drew, give up on her. She has so much kidney damage she will never get well."
>
> Although my progress seemed painfully slow, I began to improve and after six months I was nearly free of pain. Though I was weak, I was able to walk with only a slight limp.
>
> Within a few years, I was able to study Osteopathy and now, after 20 years, I am living a happy and useful life.

After rereading this wonderful letter, Dr. Charley came to a firm decision. He must do everything within his power to help his father's school continue to produce well-trained doctors for the Osteopathic profession.

Although he didn't feel the desire to do much for a while, he hoped that before long he would be able to help again. He planned to start attending state and national Osteopathic conventions and meeting with alumni and expressing his wish that the divisiveness that followed the January meeting be put to rest. With a fresh start, the college could work its way through this period without any long-term damage. He vowed to do this and eliminate his feelings of bitterness.

In the early spring, Gladys and her mother returned to Kirksville. Unfortunately, their stay in Texas had not done much to improve Gladys's condition.

The one recommended treatment for tuberculosis at the time was to move the patient to a drier and warmer climate. Dr. Charley had earlier thought about going away from Kirksville for awhile to let the dust settle, but until Gladys' return, he had about decided to stay in town, remaining in the background for a while. Now a decision was made to move to the Southwest so their daughter would be away from Kirksville before the cold weather set in. Since the other two children were attending high school and elementary school, the family planned to leave for Alamogordo, New Mexico on the thirtieth of August.

As Anna Still prepared to close their lovely home for an indefinite period, she could not help but reminisce about the many alumni and distinguished guests they had entertained, how her daughters had hosted dances, and how some of the sororities had used their dance floor. Truly their home had been a beehive of social activities. She wondered if they would ever enjoy their home in that capacity again. There was a lot of work to do to close the home before they left for New Mexico.

When the date of their leaving was announced, the townspeople of Kirksville decided they would put on the biggest going away party the town had ever seen. Nearly everyone wanted to honor the popular former mayor and longtime vice president of ASO. They also wanted to honor Anna Still, who had been so active helping her husband and participating in social and charitable activities. In addition, young Gladys was admired by many who wished her a speedy recovery.

The party was so large that the front lawn was used to accommodate the hundreds who attended. It was also the first party where individuals from both sides of the controversy mingled together in wishing the best for Dr. Charley's family, and the hope that, with Gladys recovered, they would be returning soon.

The outpouring of love, affection, and heartfelt wishes carried over for some time. Nevertheless, as Anna Still locked the house for the last time and she and her husband walked down the steps to the car, they both looked at their home with tears in their eyes. With a last wave to friends, they headed down the driveway toward what they hoped would be a temporary home in the West.

Chapter Eighteen

S THEY DROVE AWAY FROM KIRKSVILLE in their Pierce Arrow touring car, the family continued to feel the warmth of all the love and friendship so many people gave them during their send-off party. Even the dusty bumpy roads could not dim the glow. The family made frequent stops as it traveled through western Missouri, Kansas, Oklahoma, and Texas. Dr. Charley and Anna were thrilled and pleased when local Osteopaths came to visit them in their hotels whenever they stopped en route to their destination in New Mexico.

In western Texas and eastern New Mexico, where there were fewer towns, the Stills often stayed with farm families. Eating their meals with the farmers and the farmhands at large kitchen tables was fun for the children. They were excited when they drove through a large Apache Indian Reservation.

New Mexico had been a state for only six years when the family made it their home, so the youngest member of the family, Charley, hoped there were still famous gunmen walking the streets with their guns on their hips. When he found out this wasn't so, he was quite disappointed. Then when the family moved into a residence on a street named New York Avenue, his lingering illusions about the Wild West dissolved completely.

Alamogordo was a friendly town and the family was soon accepted by the local people. Elizabeth started high school and proved to be such a good basketball player that she was instrumental in helping the school's team win some games against their fiercest rivals. Dr. Charley would often squeeze the entire team into the Pierce Arrow and drive the girls to their out-of-town games.

In the meantime, Gladys seemed to be improving although somewhat slowly. She even gained back some of her lost weight. When summer arrived, the family moved up into the mountains near Cloudcroft where Gladys continued to improve. Anna began to feel that her daughter's health was so much better, perhaps they could actually consider returning to Kirksville. She was anxious to see how her home was surviving this long period of being unoccupied. However, the family decided to stay in New Mexico another year to ensure a more complete recovery for Gladys.

Dr. Charley was once again more like the normal outgoing person he used to be. Both he and Anna found new friends in "Alamo," as the locals called their town. The only indications that he had not forgotten his dismissal from ASO were his reluctance to discuss an early return to Kirksville while the controversy was still going on, and his reluctance to read anything about the school in the Kirksville newspaper to which they had subscribed. He needed to let his wounds heal a bit more before he directed his attention to what was happening at ASO. In another year he might be ready to make another significant contribution to Osteopathic education.

Many of Elizabeth's friends were entering New Mexico State University at Las Cruces for their freshman year, so she too enrolled. Gladys, who had been engaged to an Army pilot, again started talking about wedding plans. Everything seemed to be going along much better. Then the cleaning lady brought her young son to work one day. The boy had mumps and the weakened Gladys contracted the contagious disease. Within ten days, she had a massive intestinal hemorrhage and passed away.

Dr. Charley, who had been making a good recovery from his personal emotional stresses, felt this was the final blow. To lose his dear and attractive daughter who had shown so much promise in college just as she was apparently on the road to recovery left him devastated and feeling useless and unable to face the future.

The family's train ride back to Missouri with Gladys's body was the lowest and saddest period they had ever faced. After Gladys's funeral, Anna and Dr. Charley stayed at the sanatorium in Macon for the next ten months, rarely going out or visiting anyone. They also stayed completely away from Kirksville. They showed no interest in how their home was holding up. They paid no attention to the operation of ASO. Nor were they interested in whether or not Dr. George Still, by then named president of ASO, was doing a good job in that post.

Daughter Elizabeth had hurried back to New Mexico as soon as the funeral was over to complete her first year in college. Charley, Jr., was sent to Kirksville so he could again attend Benton Elementary School. He stayed at his Uncle Harry's home and shared a bedroom with his cousin Richard.

Without returning to Kirksville, Dr. Charley, Anna, and son Charley moved to La Jolla, California toward the end of August 1920 and rented a beach house. Elizabeth, who had stayed with friends in Las Cruces during the summer, was accompanied by several of them when she drove the Pierce Arrow to California so it would be available for her parents. Following a brief reunion, she returned to New Mexico for her sophomore year of college.

Anna Still, as did the wives of Andrew and Abraham before her, took over the management of the family and all its financial obligations. Dr. Charley in the meantime spent his days walking along the beach, rarely speaking to anyone.

After a year in La Jolla, the family moved to Los Angeles because, at that time, there was no high school in the beach town for Charley, Jr., to attend. He had graduated from the Kirksville elementary school. With both children in school – Elizabeth had transferred to the University of Southern California, and Charley, Jr., had enrolled at the University High School – Anna tried to convince her husband that he could no longer spend his life wandering aimlessly around the streets of Los Angeles.

Nothing had brought Charley relief from his depressed state. If it hadn't been for Dr. Will Laughlin's enthusiasm and persistence, it is hard to tell when or if this depression might have lifted.

When Dr. Will left his teaching post at ASO, he established a busy practice and felt he needed a good Osteopath to help him. He insisted that Dr. Charley had too much talent to waste just walking the streets. He told him, "You can treat a few of my patients. I will only give you the ones who don't require a lot of talking."

For nearly six months, Dr. Charley resisted. He tried talking Dr. Will into leaving him alone and letting him just stay at home. But the persistent Dr. Will drove by the house every morning and – at least at first – literally dragged Dr. Charley to the office with him. Then after about six months, Dr. Will's reluctant helper began to show signs of looking forward to going to the office and not only treating patients, but talking to them as well.

By late spring of 1922, Dr. Charley was beginning to regain quite a bit of confidence. He could talk to people again without any trouble. And once his work with patients began to bring in some income again, he developed quite a different attitude. For nearly three years, Anna had been giving him an allowance and now with spending money in his pocket – money that he earned – life seemed a lot better.

He had tried to remove himself completely from school affairs in Kirksville. But he knew that his brother-in-law, Dr. George Laughlin, probably at the urging of his wife Blanche, had applied for a license to start a competing school of Osteopathy in Kirksville. Dr. Charley and his brother Harry had agreed that if Dr. George Laughlin had any trouble borrowing enough money to finance the school, they would co-sign his loan application.

The brothers had borrowed a large sum of money from a Saint Louis bank to start the Still-Hildreth Sanatorium earlier and had been able to pay it back in a very short time. As a result, they had gained a good financial reputation.

As plans for Laughlin's new school unfolded, Dr. Charley realized that he was not yet ready to become directly involved. But he did feel ready enough to meet with other Osteopaths, so he attended the 1922 California State Convention, the first convention he had gone to since, what was for him, the ill-fated National Convention in 1917.

Another year of working with the enthusiastic Dr. Will gave Charley the strength and confidence he needed to plan his future. During the fall of 1922 and spring of 1923, he found that he once more enjoyed being with people. He was again able to keep in touch with events at ASO and have an interest in the progress of Dr. George Laughlin's new school founded earlier in 1922.

His resolve to contribute to the preservation of Osteopathic education in Kirksville was now restored. He was ready to put his shoulder to the wheel once more. In early June of 1923, the Still family once more climbed into the Pierce Arrow – repainted red to replace its original black finish – and headed for Missouri, traveling by way of Yellowstone Park. It had been nearly five years since their departure from Kirksville. Sadly, there were now only four moving back into the family home.

There was much to do to restore the house to its previous condition. Except for the few times it had been opened to clean and make minor repairs, the house that had been built for the man aspiring to be president of the college had remained closed. Once Anna had the house returned to running order, it was quickly reinstated in its role as the hub of community social activities – club meetings, sorority dances, and large dinner parties with many distinguished guests.

Dr. Charley received a warm welcome from the townspeople. He was also greeted heartily by the board and faculty of the new college. Dr. George Laughlin had stated many times that he didn't want to be in the school business, and he was certainly glad to have his brother-in-law back and contributing to the success of the new school. But he might never admit it. Even though he listened to advice, he rarely asked for it.

Dr. George Laughlin had added Dr. Harry to his board of directors shortly after he opened the A. T. Still College of Osteopathy and Surgery, named in tribute to the Old Doctor who founded the original school. He was pleased when Dr. Charley also agreed to accept an appointment to the board and to be available for advice as requested.

With the help of these two who had spent years steering the first school of Osteopathy through its growing pains and several critical periods, Dr. George Laughlin felt he had added seasoned associates who shared his commitment to sound Osteopathic education.

Dr. Charley was pleased that his brother-in-law had assembled a strong faculty steeped in fundamental Osteopathy. He was also impressed that the new school was operating on a sound financial basis, one that would help assure its stability. The fact that it was being set up to become a nonprofit institution in the near future represented some of the ideas that he had been working on for ASO when he was so abruptly fired.

As far as ASO was concerned, he had mixed emotions. He naturally felt a certain sense of loyalty to the school he had guided for nearly twenty-five years. Although its enrollment was holding up fairly well, he had talked with some alumni whose sons and daughters now attended ASO and who felt the quality of education was not as good as they would have liked. There were also reliable reports that the financial condition of ASO had been deteriorating for some time.

Dr. Charley was definitely committed to promoting good Osteopathic education, but he wanted sincerely to keep himself removed from the bitter rivalry between the two schools. So, after first offering to be an advisor, he then joined the faculty of Dr. George Laughlin's school, the A. T. Still College of Osteopathy.

With so much space now available in his home, Dr. Charley filled the extra rooms with students. Sometimes he used treating tables on the second floor to demonstrate techniques for students who often represented both colleges.

Once he settled into his new life-style, he began to think about owning show animals again. His Jersey herd had been sold years before and he had a strong desire to have livestock once more. He purchased a few Duroc Jersey pigs. In the meantime, Dr. George Laughlin had purchased some Berkshire hogs and the two men entertained themselves by discussing the merits of the two breeds. They also had an occasional discussion regarding the operation of the new college and their recommendations for improving it.

It was certainly more pleasant to talk about show animals than to plod through the myriad of problems involved in the college. However, for the first time Dr. Charley felt that he could be a more useful contributor to Osteopathic education and the profession in general without ever holding the position of college president. Now he could be free to do some teaching, show his "red pigs" at state and national swine shows, and begin a book about his father's life.

The loss of his daughter was still hard for him to bear. But having his emotional strength back, he felt ready to enter another productive period of his life. He was happy that his wife, Anna, was also making such a successful adjustment to their new life together. After having accepted so much responsibility for so long, she now seemed to be enjoying their fresh life-style.

His family was in California when Dr. George Still met his untimely death in an accident. Dr. Charley was faced with the fact that now he and his cousin would never have the opportunity to work out the divisiveness and bitterness that followed Dr. Charley's being ousted from the college and Dr. George's being named ASO president.

However, Dr. Charley felt quite a bit different about Mrs. Hamilton. Mainly, he was puzzled and disappointed. In the past, when he and her husband had met in the Hamilton home to discuss problems at the school, she had often felt free to join in their conversations. She also knew of Charley's deep commitment to the operation of the school and how he had been able to manage the college during some very difficult times. Charley had always welcomed her suggestions and she had never given him any reason to believe she was dissatisfied with his performance. She had truly dropped a bombshell when she threw her support to George Still. The scars that resulted never totally healed for Dr. Charley.

For a short period following Dr. George Still's death, ASO was run by his father, Dr. S. S. Still. The original school's financial condition continued to worsen and there was a major need to eliminate the divisiveness and to have one single school of Osteopathy in Kirksville. A resolution to the problem came in March of 1924 when Dr. George Laughlin purchased the ASO stock. On June 2 that summer, he consolidated the two institutions. Dr. Laughlin's board by then had three members of the Old Doctor's immediate family as members: Blanche Still Laughlin and her brothers, Dr. Harry and Dr. Charley.

Viewing all consolidation problems from the sidelines, Dr. Charley felt content to sit back and let his brother-in-law accept the major portion of the responsibility. He was comfortable in his new role. It allowed him to do such a variety of interesting things while making a continuing contribution to the future of Osteopathy without the day-to-day challenges of operating the school. He and Anna could do all the entertaining they both so enjoyed. And they could travel if they wished.

He could continue to dabble in raising livestock. His Duroc Jersey hogs were being shown at major State Fairs and he proved once more that he was an outstanding judge of livestock when, competing with some of the nation's wealthier Duroc owners, he won a grand championship with Wave Beauty, a perfectly proportioned Duroc sow, at the National Swine Show in Springfield, Illinois.

CHARLEY HAD NEVER THOUGHT MUCH about a career in politics, though he had enjoyed two terms as mayor of Kirksville, so it was on the spur of the moment that he registered to run for state representative from Adair County on the Republican ticket. Without doing any campaigning, he was only mildly surprised when he was elected.

He served with so much distinction that after four terms the Democrats asked if they could put him on their ticket, too. The next time he returned to Jefferson City, he had more Democratic votes than from his own party. During the sixteen years he represented Adair County, he served as chairman of several of the most important committees and was a great help to the Osteopathic profession by acting as chairman of the Health Committee several times.

The Osteopaths in Jefferson City expressed their pleasure over his work by naming the Osteopathic hospital in their city the Charles E. Still Hospital. This was indeed an honor.

The chairman of the State Republican Committee, noting Charley's popularity, asked him to run for Lieutenant Governor. Because of his age and the rigors of campaigning, Dr. Charley decided he would continue to serve as the Representative from Adair County instead.

He felt a great sense of pride when a Democratic governor chose him and his wife to be the official hosts in the Missouri Building at both the New York and San Francisco World Fairs.

He was also extremely pleased when, in the fall of 1929, his daughter, Elizabeth, and son, Charley Jr., enrolled in the Osteopathic college in Kirksville. By this time it was called the Kirksville College of Osteopathy and Surgery.

CHARLEY HAD SO MUCH TO BE PROUD OF during his lifetime, but he and his wife concluded that a high point for them was the faith that his father, Andrew – the Old Doctor – had shown in him when he was sent out as the first person besides Andrew to carry the banner of Osteopathy into a not-too-friendly world.

He remembered the day he had joined his sister and brothers to stand beside his father's chair as the statue of the Old Doctor was unveiled. They shared in the pleasure and honor of having young Charley pull the cord to unveil and reveal the wonderful sculpture.

Dr. Charley could see the gentle smile on his father's face. He knew that Andrew enjoyed the ceremony that had brought hundreds of former students – his "children," he called them – back to Kirksville to honor the Old Doctor's accomplishments. The speaker reminded the crowd that less than twenty-five years earlier, starting from a small frame building "right there" a block away, Dr. Andrew T. Still's profession of healing was first recognized. Further, he said, in the subsequent years this special science developed by Andrew had been introduced internationally, circling the globe. He noted that Osteopathy graduates were currently serving in every state of the Union.

Andrew's children could see the pleasure these statements brought him. As his eyes had lit up, they all felt the thrill of this momentous occasion and were grateful they had had the privilege of having Andrew with them for this celebration.

While Andrew had been wheeled back from the front yard to his home, the crowd had stood waiting for a final wave from the Old Doctor. With some assistance, he climbed to his feet and feebly raised his arm in a farewell gesture.

As Andrew had disappeared through the front door, it had been obvious to Dr. Charley that his father would not be with him much longer. Over the years, when he had accepted much of the responsibility for the operation of the school, it had always been helpful to have his father to talk to when major problems arose.

For a moment he felt quite alone as he contemplated the future. It would be difficult, he realized, to keep Osteopathy a separate system of therapy and to keep ASO in the forefront of Osteopathic education without the Old Doctor's direct influence.

This would be his challenge. Dr. Charley knew he would need all the help he could get, along with Divine guidance.

FOR THE NEXT TWENTY-SEVEN YEARS, Dr. Charley was happy that he was physically able to attend every board meeting. Although he gave much of his time to the college and his profession, he was also pleased that he could serve the people of Missouri in the legislature.

Dr. Charley was a legislator for sixteen years and rarely missed a committee meeting or regular session. He gained the reputation for fair-mindedness and for considering the people first whenever he cast his votes on political issues.

During their years in Jefferson City, Dr. Charley and Ann became popular and admired figures. It was a great loss to all when, in December of 1943, after a long illness, Dr. Charley's helpmate of over fifty years passed away.

Perhaps one thing that endeared him to the other legislators was the farewell dinner that he gave members of the Senate and House each year when legislative sessions ended. His party had become one of the outstanding social events in Jefferson City.

As Dr. Charley entered his eighties, the steps of the capitol seemed to have gotten steeper. Since he hated to use the service elevator, he finally had to have what was to be a truly final farewell dinner. Back in Kirksville, however, he continued to attend college board meetings until the fall of 1952.

At this time, Dr. Charley entered a nursing home. For a short while the president and secretary of the board would take a tape recorder to his room before each board meeting and would record his suggestions and thoughts regarding the administrative operations of the Kirksville College of Osteopathy and Surgery. Although his body was feeble, he was able to think clearly, and because of his great love for his profession and years of experience, he offered viable suggestions.

In May of 1955, Dr. Charley was now nearly ninety years old. The college president and secretary of the board made one last visit to record his thoughts. In early July, 1955, Dr. Charley passed away.

ANDREW AND HIS ELDEST SON, CHARLEY, had, for nearly all the years of their adult lives, dedicated themselves to seeing that the values of this new profession would not be lost and that humanity would benefit from the discovery and development of Osteopathy by these two devoted pioneering doctors.

NOTES

I must congratulate my father for providing so much material in his notes on his father's life as well as on the early history of the school and the profession. No one was in a better position to chronicle the events so well. I hope I have properly used his notes, his collection of letters, and our personal conversations, to give an accurate picture of the life and times of Andrew Still and his family.

Perhaps the most fitting tribute to my father, Dr. Charles E. Still, was this one written by Dr. Englehard, D.O. It appeared in the November, 1936 issue of the *Journal of Osteopathy* under the headline, "Missouri Association Honors Founder's Son: Presents Life Membership on 'Dr. Charley Day.'" I include it in its entirety here.

Dr. Charley, as we love to call him, is known all over this country by that kindly name, had grave responsibilities, for they had undertaken a herculean task of founding a science of healing in opposition to the American Medical teaching, and founding a school to teach this new science, Osteopathy, without chart or compass to guide them was a leap into the unknown. It took determination and perseverance and imagination to carry them through. Only a dreamer with a vision impelling him onward could have succeeded with the undertaking.

To build buildings, secure teachers, establish a curriculum and see that no false teaching was given, all multiplied their task. Sometimes, like the French Government, nearly the whole cabinet of teachers had to be dismissed in one way or another, for medical men as teachers knew the text-book but did not have the vision of Osteopathy and could not teach the ideas of the founder. These and many others arose, recognition by the Legislature, etc. Dr. Charley as acting head of the Board was busy on all these questions. Decisions had to be made and thanks to their caution and devotion to the good of the school, their decisions were sound and worked out for the final victory of Osteopathy.

Strong opposition and force was brought to bear on the subject of what should be taught in the school. In the early days, many advisors insisted that a medical course be added to the curriculum being deluded by the claims of medicine and not understanding or realizing that Osteopathy is Nature's own way to health. But Dr. A. T. Still and Dr. Charley were in control and so the curriculum remained clear and the teaching that the primary and great cause of disease is faulty body mechanics and that the body is supplied with all the necessary chemicals was continued.

Can you imagine what would have happened to our profession if the founders of the first school had yielded in those early days to the misguided advocates of medicine? If Dr. Charley and his father had not stood firmly on the conviction of what should be taught in the school that we would not have an independent osteopathic school in the land today. So therefore, we owe to Dr. Charley more than to any other living man, our gratitude and appreciation for the fight he made for twenty-five years, yea, twenty-five long years, to guide the school to success and victory over its enemies who would have destroyed it in its early life.

Why do I love to honor Dr. Charley? For many years he was not only the vice-president of the Board of Directors of the school but one of the most successful practitioners of Osteopathy and was my family physician and later my instructor. He taught us to make a thorough diagnosis, for he said then you have your patients half cured to begin with. He is my friend and your friend. Few, if any, in our profession have more friends than Dr. Charley, for he is a friend to us all and we all love him in return.

Why do we honor Dr. Charley today? For his part in developing Osteopathy and for his life of usefulness and unselfishness and the good he had done and is doing. His work is not finished. He is not charged with the responsibilities of the school now but his presence goes far to build good will and fellowship and keep up the traditions of the school. Who better than Dr. Charley can hand down to this generation and the students in our schools today, the real truths taught by the 'Old Doctor'? Who can recount the story of the life of Dr. Still better than Dr. Charley? It is good to see Dr. George Laughlin, who is now carrying the banner of the school, walking arm in arm, as it were, with the hero of this hour, for we know they are carrying on and teaching the everlasting principles of Osteopathy.

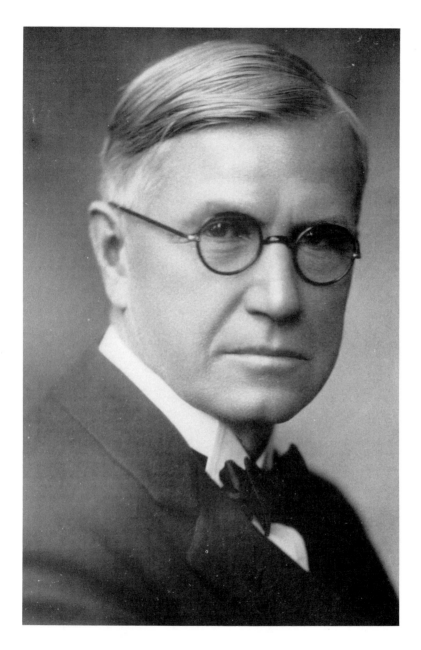

Charles E. Still, Missouri State Representative

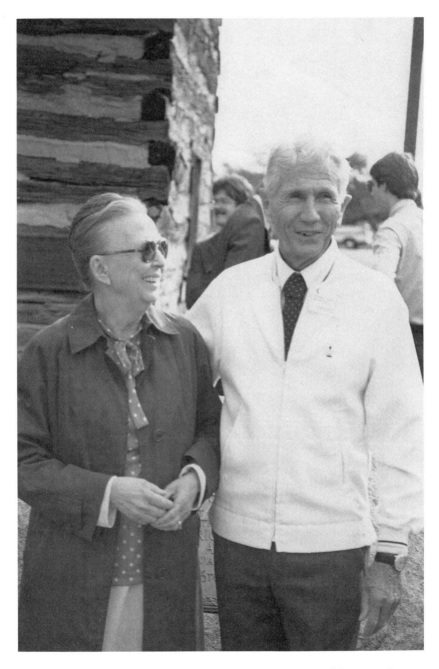

Charles E. Still, Jr., and his cousin, Mary Jane Laughlin Denslow

Epilogue

Y STRETCHING MY MEMORY to its farthest point, I can vaguely remember some things that occurred in 1912. From 1913 on things are much clearer and I hope that my recall from then on hasn't been too faulty.

I have been asked many times, "Do you remember your grandfather?" Since I was ten years and eight months old when he died, and he lived right next door, I certainly remember him well, in about the same way that any ten-year-old boy would remember a grandparent who lived nearby.

The next question I have been asked is, "What do you most remember about him?" I think the thing I remember most is that he was the only person I ever saw walking with a staff. The fact that he wore his heavy clothes year around also impressed me. One of my early memories of him is that, while he was still taking his walks, not only did he always wear boots, but he rarely put both pants legs into them. I suppose earlier he tucked his pants into his boots, but in later years there was usually one pants leg flapping out in a most inelegant manner.

I have also been asked if he was a loving grandfather. I have always doubted that he really noticed me much. There were a few times when I tried to perform some simple athletic stunt that probably made him wonder how a grandson of his could have been so lacking in coordination.

We did have one thing in common: a love of freshly baked pies. Aunt Blanche Laughlin had a cook who could really bake wonderful fruit pies and cream pies. There were several times when Grandfather Still and I spent what seemed to be forever waiting for the pies to cool enough so that we could sample them.

I had been told by my parents that my grandfather was a very important man. They also told me that quite a few famous people came to visit him. In nice weather, I would meander over and listen to their conversations on his front porch for a while. Frankly, state governors, congressmen, and United States senators didn't impress me. Even well-known writers and musicians didn't impress me much.

My attitude changed rather significantly, however, when William "Buffalo Bill" Cody came to Kirksville with his Wild West Show and spent nearly an hour with grandfather on the front porch in earnest conversation. Buffalo Bill was a real hero of mine at that time and from then on I had a great deal more respect and admiration for my grandfather.

Looking back on that occasion, it may have been what the local newspaper said: "It was a day that no matter how long 'Little Charley' lives, it would be a day he would never forget."

After Cody's visit, and when they had a chance to reminisce about the fact that his father and my grandfather had served in the Kansas Territorial Legislature during those turbulent pre-War times, Buffalo Bill came to our house. As a surprise, Mother had prepared an early lunch during which I got to sit next to my hero. This was followed by an invitation to be his special guest at the afternoon performance of his Wild West Show. He introduced me to many of the cast and to two or three real Indian chiefs.

From that time on, I rarely failed to check on grandfather's front porch visitors.

Another high point in my early life occurred during the unveiling ceremonies for Grandfather Still's statue. Since I was the youngest grandson at that time, I was elected to pull the cord at the unveiling ceremonies. They did not inform me of this important assignment in advance, but it was reported that I did a credible job.

Sixty-nine years later, after his statue had been refinished from years of being exposed to the weather, I was once again selected to pull the cord during the second unveiling. I didn't do it as efficiently as I had the first time, at age ten.

I was too young to remember much about my father's outstanding Jersey cattle, but by the time he was raising Duroc hogs, I certainly had the opportunity to be exposed to, and to learn quite a bit about, what makes a quality show animal. I must have been a slow learner, because Dad often said of me, "For a lad who has literally been raised with red pigs, he knows less about them than anyone I know."

The year that we won the grand championship at the national show in Illinois, I knew that my Dad had high hopes for his entry. When I saw that our sow was not placed in line at the final judging, which was the usual procedure, I was beginning to feel sorry for him. Finally, I turned to some of the knowledgeable spectators and said, "I thought our entry had a good chance and they haven't even placed her in line."

After some discussion, they replied, condescendingly, "Your sow is so good that she had won even before the competition started."

From the time I was seven and until my tenth birthday, I had the privilege of serving as the mascot for both ASO football and baseball teams. Since the teams had no official symbol and were usually referred to as just "the Osteopaths" or by out-of-town newspapers as the "Kirksville Osteopaths," I suppose it was proper for me to have that role. It was several years later that the teams began to be called the Rams.

During football season, I was only allowed to sit on the bench. However, during the baseball season, I had the opportunity to play catch with some of the players.

The highlight of my career as mascot occurred during my last year of service when, in a game between the faculty and the regular team, I was allowed to be a "pinch runner" for the varsity. I was so excited that after I took my place on third base the coach had to take time to be sure that I knew where home plate was located.

In the late 1930s, after I had been in practice for three or four years, I dropped into the office of one of the former baseball players during a visit to the Los Angeles area. He was by then a most successful practitioner with a spacious office and several assistants. There must have been nearly a hundred patients waiting to be treated.

Within a few seconds after I told the receptionist who I was, a booming voice over the intercom announced, "Send in the mascot."

I felt all eyes riveted on me as I was led sheepishly back to receive a warm welcome from one of my former baseball idols. I didn't feel nearly as mature, or professional, as I had when I first entered the office. I now had a new role – that of "ex-mascot."

Seriously speaking, for the several thousand like myself who practiced manipulative Osteopathy for years without the aid of drugs or antibiotics and successfully treated a variety of acute infections, did we in some way either free up or stimulate the immune system so that it could better the body's ability to resist infection? Why has not more effort been made to research why and how manipulation apparently improved such a variety of serious infections? Was Andrew Still really being facetious in saying that there is no such thing as disease – only the inability of an individual's body to resist infection?

While medical science finds more and more so-called diseases, while viruses change from year to year, and drugs and antibiotics lose their effectiveness, maybe it is about time to research any avenue that might lead us to a way to stimulate the body's immune system to more effectively resist infection.

In conclusion, I am proud that I finally got around to writing about the lives of some truly interesting and exciting people. I am even prouder that I am fortunate enough to be related to them and am happy that I knew so many of them personally.

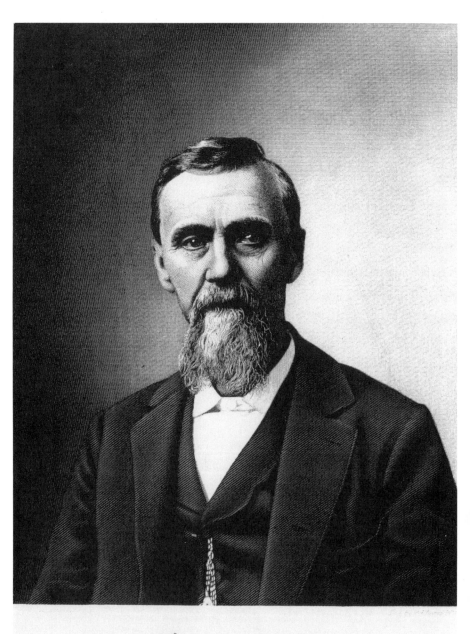

Kindly yours—

Andrew T. Still.

Index